THE MIND GUT CONNECTION

The Path to Inner Harmony Strengthening Clarity, Confidence, and Balance in Your Life

CHERISH DUTRO

CONTENTS

BONUS WORKBOOK

www.Dutro-Publishing.com

INTRODUCTION: THE WHISPERING WISDOM OF OUR SECOND BRAIN

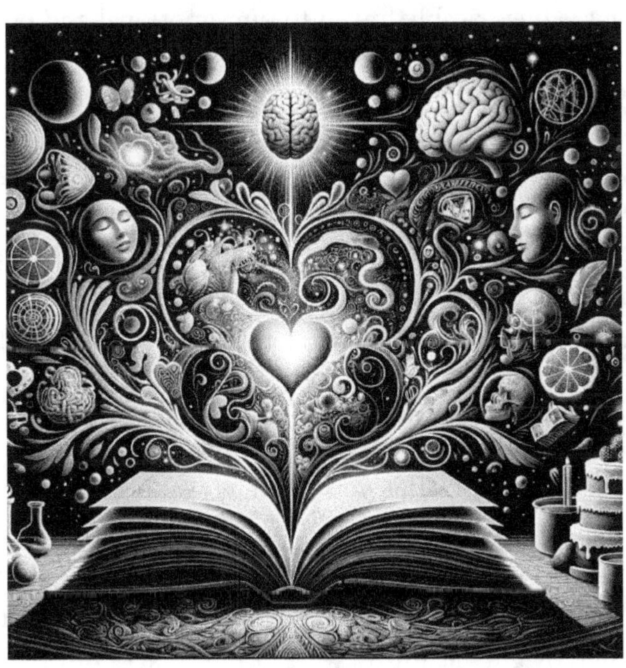

Have you ever had a hunch so palpable that it felt like an unseen force nudging you toward an unknown destiny? Strap in because I'm about to take you on a whirlwind tour of those sensations. Picture this: a crossroads moment, logic tugging you one way, but your gut? It's practically hollering in the opposite direction. Heeding that call didn't just tweak my life's trajectory; it catapulted me into the enthralling world where our guts and minds waltz in unspoken harmony.

This book, my friends, is my heart—and gut—a labor of love. It unfurls the thesis that the mind-gut connection isn't just fascinating; it's the secret sauce to unlocking a life brimming with vitality and serenity. Forget about passing on that extra slice of cake out of fear for your tummy; we're diving headfirst into how our gut's well-being is inextricably linked to our emotional and psychological fabric.

Crafted to whisk you away on a journey from the scientific underpinnings of the mind-gut concord to actionable nuggets of wisdom for cherishing this delicate bond, this tome aims to enlighten and equip. Prepare to gobble up (pun very much intended) knowledge that will empower you to turn your gut into a stalwart ally in your quest for emotional balance and mental clarity.

Through my escapades sailing the turbulent seas of gut health and mental equilibrium, I offer you a unique vantage point peppered with a healthy dose of humor and sprinkled with empathy, particularly for my comrades in the golden years. My narrative, enriched with personal tales and a smidge of wit, shines a spotlight on the significance of gut health as we gracefully age, resonating with your most profound queries and reflections.

Woven with engaging stories and life lessons, this book is akin to a cozy chat over a cup of tea, simplifying the complex interplay of science in the mind-gut dialogue into enjoyable, easy-to-swallow nuggets of wisdom, leaving you not only informed but inspired to nurture a healthier relationship with your body.

THE GUT-BRAIN AXIS: NATURE'S GOSSIP LINE

In the wee hours of the morning, when the world is as quiet as a mouse and seems to be holding its breath, there's an elderly gentleman in my neighborhood who's out in his garden. He's not just puttering around for the sake of it; oh no, he's knee-deep in an activity as old as time itself. With every seed he tucks into the soil and every pesky weed, he shows the door, he's partaking in a ritual that goes beyond the garden fence. This gardening lark, you see, is a bit like tending to the bustling city of microbes residing in our guts. Most folks don't give a second thought to these microscopic inhabitants, but they're as busy as bees, playing a starring role in our health, mood, and choices at the buffet table. This chapter pulls back the curtain on the gut-brain axis, the invisible wire that ties our tummies to our noggin, and how this bit of magic could turn the health world on its head.

At the core of this intriguing natter (also known as a conversation) between our gut and brain is a cosmopolitan, two-way street known as the gut-brain axis. This network is like the town gossip, constantly exchanging juicy tidbits influencing our bellies' feel and our overall zest for life and ability to dodge illnesses.

BIOLOGICAL BASIS

To get a handle on this chit-chat, we need to introduce the leading players: the central nervous system (CNS), the enteric nervous system (ENS), and the bustling metropolis of microbes that call our gut home, collectively known as the microbiota. The CNS, comprising the brain and spinal cord, has a natter with the ENS, affectionately dubbed the "second brain," through a hotline known as the vagus nerve. This nerve is the gossip column of the body, passing whispers back and forth between the brain's ivory tower and the gut's winding streets.

Our gut's residents, including a cast of trillions of bacteria, viruses, and fungi, join the conversation with the CNS and ENS, churning out all sorts of substances that can sway brain function. They're like the local moonshiners, producing neurotransmitters such as serotonin, which is crucial for keeping our spirits up and is brewed up in the gut, not the brain, as you might expect.

Historical Perspective

The buzz about the gut-brain axis marks a seismic shift in how we think about our insides. For donkey's years, the gut and brain were considered distant relatives at best, with their interactions chalked up to nothing more than the rumbles and grumbles of hunger and fullness. This old-school view started to get a facelift with some pioneering studies in the early 20th century. Still, until the glitzy era of modern genetic sequencing, scientists could get nosy about the gut microbiome's role in our health and happiness.

This field has been like a gold rush, uncovering treasures about how our gut's microbial mix can touch everything from autoimmune conditions to the mysteries of the mind. The revelation that our microbiota can chinwag with the brain has smudged the lines between different branches of science, ushering in a more rounded approach to keeping ourselves in tip-top shape.

Health Implications

The chitter-chatter between our gut and brain has big-time implications for our well-being. A mix-up in the gut's microbial community has been linked to a variety of ailments, from the tummy troubles of irritable bowel syndrome (IBS) to heftier issues like obesity and even brainy concerns like Alzheimer's and Parkinson's. Plus, this gut-brain hotline is crucial in managing the body's stress response, with too much worry known to poke holes in our gut barrier, leading to what the layman calls "leaky gut."

This ongoing natter also has a say in our mood. The up-and-coming field of psychobiotics is looking at how certain friendly bacteria might boost our mental health by tweaking the gut-brain axis. By adjusting the volume of gut bacteria's chatter, it's possible to influence the production of neurotransmitters that regulate our mood, opening up new paths for tackling gloom and anxiety without relying solely on the medicine cabinet.

FUTURE DIRECTIONS

As we tiptoe into new territories, the research into the gut-brain axis is brimming with potential. Cutting-edge studies are sizing how our microbiota's unique makeup can affect our disease risk and how we react to treatments, laying the groundwork for bespoke medical strategies that could cook up interventions based on our gut's personal recipe.

Let's spill the tea on the non-stop chinwag between our gut and brain. They're old friends, constantly gossiping away beneath our notice. They communicate through a complex network of chemical signals and neural pathways, which, believe it or not, play a massive part in how chipper or gloomy we feel, how we handle stress, and even in the choices we make at the dinner table. Getting the hang of tuning into this internal dialogue can be a game-changer, giving us the scoop on managing stress, picking the grub that makes us feel grand, and keeping our spirits high.

Chemical Gossip

Imagine your gut as a chatty Cathy, nattering away to your brain using a cocktail of neurotransmitters and hormones. Many of these chemical signals are the same as the ones buzzing around in our central nervous system (CNS). Take serotonin, the so-called 'happy chemical,' a big deal for keeping our mood sunny. Would you believe about 90% of it is whipped up in our gut? Then there's gamma-aminobutyric acid (GABA), which keeps our nerves from fraying, and glutamate, which keeps our thinking cap in tip-top shape. These chemicals are the gut's way of dropping a line to the brain, affecting how we feel from one moment to the next.

Neural Chatter

The main gossip line between the gut and brain is the vagus nerve. This whopper of a nerve stretches from the brainstem down to the belly, passing on the latest from both ends. It's like the gut and brain are on a direct call, updating each other on the latest internal news. The enteric nervous system (ENS) in the gut, boasting over 100 million nerve cells, also gets in on the act. It can run the show in the gut but keeps the brain in the loop.

Mind Matters

The back-and-forth between our gut and brain has a hefty say in how we feel upstairs. A tummy full of trouble, with the wrong kind of bacteria taking over, might start churning out nasties that can fog up our brain, leading to mood swings or the blues.

On the flip side, a gut that's in harmony can be like a cheerleader for our mental well-being, pumping out the good stuff that keeps us feeling on top of the world. And let's not forget stress—it's a two-way street with our gut. A dose of the jitters can shake up our gut flora and make our insides a bit more leaky than we'd like, showing how tight-knit the gut-brain buddy system is.

Tuning In

Getting in sync with your gut's whispers (or shouts) is a mix of gut instinct and good old-fashioned observation. Start by keeping a food diary—note what you eat and how it makes you feel. This detective work can reveal much about how your gut buddies react to different foods. Mindful eating is another key; take your time, savor your meals, and notice how they sit with you. Meditation and gentle exercises, like yoga or a stroll, can also fine-tune your gut-brain connection, helping you pick up on what your insides are trying to tell you.

Attention to these inner signals can lead to more thoughtful food choices, better stress management, and a more even-keeled mood. Noticing that a specific snack leaves you bloated or zapped of energy can steer you towards foods your gut is more in tune with. Similarly, seeing the link between stress and your digestive upsets can motivate you to embrace relaxation techniques, showcasing the deep conversation within our bodies.

The constant gab between our gut and brain is a big deal, influencing our mood, stress levels, what we eat, and even how well we fend off germs. By learning to eavesdrop on this inner dialogue, we can make moves that boost our physical health and keep our mental and emotional well-being in the pink.

1.3 TUMMY TROUBLES AND MOOD SWINGS: THE EMOTIONAL ROLLERCOASTER INSIDE US

It's quite the spectacle, the way our innards and emotions do the tango, each step and turn affecting the other in a dance so intricate it'd give the Bolshoi Ballet a run for its money. This connection is a fleeting partnership and a lifelong pas de deux between how we feel and how our gut behaves. Let's dive into the curious world of emotional digestion, or as I like to call it, "Why does my tummy turn somersaults when I'm upset?"

Emotional Tidbits

Our emotions are like puppet masters to our digestive system, pulling strings in ways both subtle and profound. Have you ever noticed how a flutter of joy can make your tummy gurgle with glee or how a wave of anxiety can send you sprinting for the nearest bathroom? That's your gut, responding in real time to your emotional rollercoaster. But the plot thickens, my friends. Our feelings do more than just stir up temporary turmoil; they can rejig the very crew of bacteria setting up shop in our gut, impacting everything from our immune defenses to our mood and even how we act. It's a feedback loop so intricate it makes the mystery of who took the last biscuit seem trivial.

Stress and Its Bellyaches

The saga of stress and digestion is a tale as old as time, with chronic stress playing the villain in dramas ranging from irritable bowel syndrome (IBS) to indigestion and constipation. When stress enters the scene, it signals for cortisol to take the stage, a hormone that, in the spotlight, can throw our gut functions into disarray, disturb our inner microbial peace, and even make our gut walls as leaky as a sieve. This can lead to a cascade of inflammation and heighten our stress, a vicious cycle that's as hard to break as my habit of sneaking chocolates before dinner.

But fear not! The story doesn't end here. Our eating patterns often bear the brunt of stress, leading us down a path of sugary and fatty temptations that only add to our gut's distress. Understanding this melodrama is the first step toward producing a more harmonious gut-brain production.

Tales of Gut Healing

Fortunately, the script isn't set in stone. There are plenty of strategies to coax our emotional and gut health back into a loving embrace:

- Mindfulness and Meditation: Like a balm to a bee sting, practices such as mindfulness can calm the stormy seas of stress, easing our digestive woes and even jazzing up the microbial party in our gut. A little daily zen can go a long way in harmonizing our internal dialogue.
- Regular Foot-Tapping and Body-Grooving: Exercise, my dears, isn't just a boon for the ticker; it's a symphony for the soul and a banquet for the belly. Whether it's a merry tour around the park, the graceful arcs of yoga, a lively jig in the privacy of your living room, or the buoyant joy of swimming and water aerobics, each form of movement has its own magic.
- Culinary Adventures: Embarking on a dietary journey filled with whole, fiber-rich foods and the tangy zest of fermented delights supports a vibrant gut flora. Steering

clear of processed, sugary, and greasy fare can also keep the peace in our belly.

- The Sweet Embrace of Slumber: Never underestimate the power of a good night's rest, especially when stress and gut troubles are afoot. Quality sleep is like a lullaby for gut microbes, soothing stress and fostering a serene belly.

The Retired Teacher's Journey

Imagine, if you will, a retired teacher. Let's call him Mr. Thompson. After decades spent in the cacophony of classrooms, his days of discipline and dedication had transitioned into a quieter existence. Yet, the echoes of stress didn't fade with the final ringing of the school bell; they morphed into a relentless companion, irritable bowel syndrome (IBS). Mr. Thompson, a man of logic and lesson plans, found himself at the mercy of his own body, with his gut playing the role of an unruly student, refusing to heed his commands.

Skepticism was his initial reaction when a friend suggested mindfulness meditation. "What does sitting quietly do with my digestive tumult?" he pondered. But, as the adage goes, desperation breeds innovation—or, in Mr. Thompson's case, a willingness to try anything. He embarked on this mindfulness journey with the same dedication he applied to his teaching, setting aside time each day to sit, breathe, and simply be.

The transformation didn't happen overnight. It was a gradual shift, like the seasons changing outside his study window. But over time, Mr. Thompson noticed something remarkable. The IBS flare-ups became less frequent, his mind felt more precise, and his sleep improved. It was as if the mindfulness practice had calmed the storm in his mind and quelled the rebellion in his gut. He found himself more in tune with his body's needs, making dietary adjustments that further eased his symptoms. Mr. Thompson's story became one of triumph, a testament to the power of mindfulness in restoring mental peace and physical harmony.

The Grandmother's Transformation

Now, let's turn our attention to a grandmother whom we'll call Mrs. Garcia. In the aftermath of her beloved partner's passing, Mrs. Garcia found herself adrift in a sea of grief. This sorrow wasn't hers to bear alone; it seeped into her very being, manifesting in digestive despair. Where once there was joy in shared meals, and the garden tended, there was now only a lingering sadness and a stomach in knots.

The suggestion to incorporate daily walks seemed too simplistic at first. What relief could a stroll through the park offer against the weight of her loss? Yet, as Mrs. Garcia began her routine, something within her shifted. The rhythm of her steps became a meditation, the fresh air a balm to her aching heart. She resumed gardening, nurturing life in the soil as a gentle reminder of nature's cycles—loss and renewal.

Her dietary habits transformed as well. Inspired by the bounty of her garden, she embraced a diet rich in fibers and fermented foods, marveling at how these changes seemed to ease her digestive issues. Over time, the walks, the gardening, and the dietary shifts wove together into a tapestry of healing. Mrs. Garcia found herself not just coping with her grief but growing through it, with her gut health mirroring this journey of recovery.

The Harmonious Opera of Life

Mr. Thompson and Mrs. Garcia's stories are more than individual anecdotes; they're stanzas in the greater opera of life, illustrating the profound interplay between our emotions and our gut health. Their experiences underscore a universal truth: we can foster dynamic equilibrium and digestive bliss by listening to and caring for our emotional selves. In the grand opera of existence, where emotions and physical health are inextricably linked, their stories serve as a potent reminder that healing, in its most holistic sense, is possible and within reach.

1.4 CHATTING UP YOUR INNER ECOSYSTEM: THE GUT-BRAIN BANTER AND YOUR MOOD

Nestled within the cozy confines of our digestive system lies a bustling metropolis far more influential than any urban sprawl: the gut microbiome. This microscopic society, teeming with bacteria, viruses, and fungi, is a testament to the wonders of the human body and a key player in the drama of our emotional well-being.

Microbiome Mingle

Think of the gut microbiome as a cocktail party in your belly, where trillions of micro-guests play their parts in keeping you hale and hearty. They're busy breaking down your dinner, whipping up vitamins, keeping the peace with pathogens, and—here's the kicker—gossiping with your brain via the gut-brain hotline. This chit-chat between your gut's inhabitants and your noggin lays down the red carpet for a fascinating field: psychobiotics. It turns out the state of this microbial shindig can swing your mood, paint your emotions, and even tinker with your mental health.

The Happiness Recipe

Diving into science is like peeling an onion of happiness, layer by fascinating layer. Some of the critters at this belly party, dubbed "psychobiotics," are busy brewing mood-modulating chemicals like serotonin and dopamine. Your gut bugs can tickle your brain's happy centers, providing a natural lift to your spirits. Moreover, a balanced guest list in your microbiome soirée can arm you against stress, turning you into an emotional ninja.

A highlight reel from research avenue has shown that tweaking this microbial mix could dial down anxiety and dim the gloom of depression, hinting at a gut makeover as a fresh path to cloud nine. This interplay between gut and gray matter opens thrilling new doors for tackling mental health, with a yogurt spoon or a fiber-rich feast as potential tools in our emotional toolkit.

Diet's Role in the Emotional Tango

Now, onto the buffet of life: our diet. What we pile on our plates can either be an RSVP to a diverse and triumphant gut party or a party pooper to our microbial harmony, with ripple effects on our mood and emotions. High-fiber fare—think fruits, veggies, and whole grains—rolls out the red carpet for beneficial bacteria, fostering a gut environment that's a beacon of balance and joy.

And let's not forget the zest of life: fermented foods. Yogurt, kefir, sauerkraut, and their cultured comrades are like the life of the party, infusing your gut with probiotics that jazz up microbial diversity and, consequently, your mood. The supporting act, prebiotics—garlic, onions, and their crunchy friends—feed the good guys, ensuring the party in your gut keeps hopping, and your mood stays buoyant.

A Spoonful of Practical Wisdom

So, how do we keep the party grooving to the beat of happiness in our gut? Here's a sprinkle of sage advice:

- **Fiber Fiesta:** Load your plate with a rainbow of fibrous foods to keep the good bacteria grooving.
- **Fermented Fun:** Invite the likes of yogurt and sauerkraut to the table regularly for a probiotic boost.
- **Prebiotic Party**: Don't skimp on garlic, onions, and their prebiotic pals to fuel the beneficial bacteria.

- **Junk Food Jail:** Keep processed munchies and sugary snacks at bay; they're party crashers to your gut bash.
- **Hydration Station**: Drink plenty of water to keep the digestive dance floor slick and the bacteria bopping.
- **Move to the Groove:** Regular exercise gets the gut party jumping, encouraging a happy microbiome mix.
- **Stress-less Soiree:** Embrace meditation, yoga, or a quiet cuppa to keep stress from spiking the punch at your gut party.

Embracing these mindful morsels of lifestyle and diet can jazz up the microbial jamboree in your gut and lift the curtain on a more emotionally harmonious you. This gut-brain banter underscores the symphony of our existence, where caring for our inner ecosystem can tune our emotional well-being to a pitch-perfect melody.

1.5 WHEN YOUR BELLY TIES KNOTS: STRESS AND THE GUT'S LOVE-HATE RELATIONSHIP

Diving into the saga of stress and our guts is like opening a book you can't put down—a tale filled with twists, turns, and a bit of science magic that's as fascinating as accurate. Picture this: stress doesn't just throw a spanner in our mental works; it waltzes right into our digestive system, setting off fireworks as it goes. And just like in any good story, our gut doesn't just sit there; it talks back, creating a loop as intricate as a dance routine in one of those old-timey musicals.

The Plot Thickens

Here's the scoop: when stress enters stage left, it's not alone. It brings along a fanfare of hormones, including our not-so-pal cortisol. This rascal has a knack for stirring the pot in our gut, changing the pace it moves, inflaming the neighborhood, and even making the walls a bit too welcoming to unwanted guests. This upheaval can leave our gut flora in disarray, leading to discomfort and even more stress, showing us just how much of a two-way street this relationship really is.

Flip the Script

But fear not, dear reader, for this tale is not without its heroes. Our trusty allies are stepping into the limelight to break this vicious cycle: diet, exercise, and the art of chilling out. A culinary cast of whole foods, fiber champions, and fermented stars support a gut flora ready to take on stress's worst. Physical activity, too, jumps in like a knight in shining armor, sweeping stress off its feet and fostering a gut microbiome as diverse as the crowd at a Beatles concert.

Remember the power of a good night's rest and finding those precious moments of peace in a day. They're like the quiet heroes, working behind the scenes to keep our microbiome in harmony and stress at bay.

The Magic of Mindfulness

Enter mindfulness and meditation, the wizards of stress reduction, wielding their power to calm the mind and, by extension, soothe the gut. Imagine taking a few minutes each day just to breathe, to be truly present with your meal, or to stretch and bend in yoga, letting the day's worries melt away like butter on hot toast.

Picture a stressed-out executive, their belly in knots over the latest board meeting. They find solace in yoga and a gut-friendly diet; lo and behold, the stress begins to ebb, and the digestive woes start to fade. Or consider the tale of a woman, her nerves frayed and her gut in rebellion, who discovers the healing power of mindfulness. Eight weeks later, she's not only calmer, but her tummy troubles have taken a backseat.

These stories aren't just heartwarming anecdotes; they're proof in the pudding (preferably a probiotic-rich one) that we can untangle the knot between stress and our guts with a sprinkle of determination and the right tools in our kit. We can chart a course toward a happier belly and a calmer mind through the magic of mindful eating, the rhythm of regular exercise, the serenity of sufficient sleep, and the quiet power of meditation. So, here's to turning the page on stress and letting our gut live happily ever after.

SUMMARY AND HOMEWORK FOR CHAPTER ONE

Let's wrap up this gardening party with a call to action that's as enriching for your gut as it is for your soul. Imagine, if you will, our elderly friend in the garden at dawn, a symbol of what we aim for a balanced, flourishing ecosystem in our gardens and within ourselves. Here's your blueprint for nurturing this inner garden, a plan to weave the wisdom of this chapter into the tapestry of your daily life:

1. Dine with Your Microbes in Mind

Just as you might choose companions who bring out the best in you, select foods that do the same for your gut. Embark on a culinary adventure with fiber-rich foods, vibrant fruits, and hearty whole grains. Invite fermented friends like yogurt and kimchi to your table often—they're not just foods but a lifeline to a happier belly.

2. Gossip with Your Gut

Learn the language of your gut. Keep a diary if it helps. Notice how it reacts to different foods, stress, and joyous moments. This isn't navel-gazing; it's about becoming fluent in the whispers and shouts of your own body, understanding its needs, and responding with care.

3. Dance, Walk, Swim—Move!

Your body craves movement like a garden craves the sun. Whether it's yoga that bends and stretches you gently into shape, a brisk walk that clears the cobwebs, or a swim that feels like a hug from the water, find the joy in moving. It's a love letter to your gut, heart, and brain.

4. Cultivate Calm

In the hustle and bustle of life, carving out moments for meditation, mindfulness, or simply sitting with a cup of tea and watching the world go by isn't laziness—it's essential maintenance. Like pruning back overgrown branches to let in the light, these practices clear our minds, soothe our guts, and prepare us for whatever the day may hold.

5. Embrace the Night

In our 24/7 world, sleep is often the first sacrifice on the altar of productivity. Reclaim it. Good sleep is the soil from which good health grows. It's when the body repairs, the mind sifts through the day, and the gut takes a deep breath and prepares for a new day.

6. Join the Conversation

Remember, the gut-brain axis is the body's internal social network, a buzzing line of communication that influences your mood, your health, and your view of the world. Engage with it, nurture it, and the conversation can be surprisingly enlightening.

7. Share Your Story

Just as our elderly neighbor shares his gardening wisdom, share what you learn about your own journey. Much like our gardens, our stories are meant to be shared—spreading seeds of knowledge and understanding that can blossom in unexpected ways.

By adopting these practices, you're not just tending to a garden of microorganisms but cultivating a life of balance, health, and joy. So, roll up your sleeves, my dear readers. It's time to tend to our inner gardens with the same love, patience, and joy as our friend in his early morning Eden. Let's grow together.

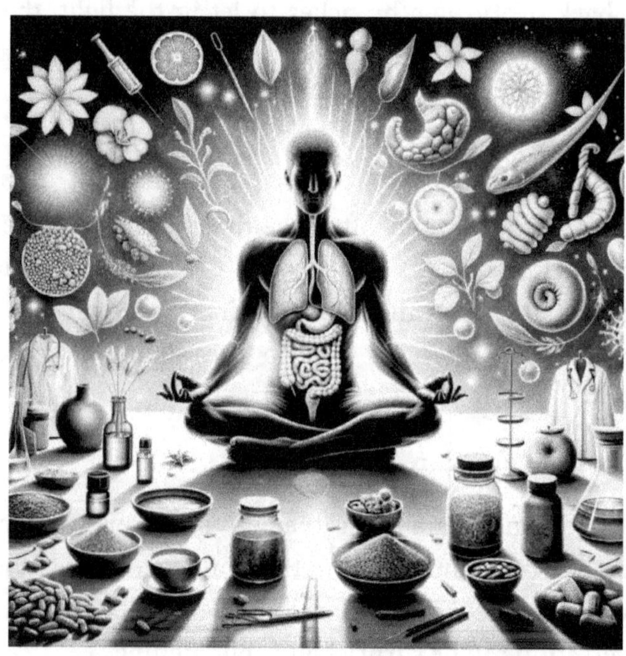

TURNING THE PAGE: KEEPING OUR INNER GARDEN FLOURISHING PAST 60

Imagine your garden, once a riot of color and life in the spring, easing into the dignified elegance of autumn. The leaves don a spectrum of reds, oranges, and yellows, each a silent testament to change. There's a certain crispness in the air, carrying tales of transformation. Much like the steadfast turn of seasons, our vessels of life—our bodies—waltz through their own seasons, with our gut playing a leading role in this dance of years. In this chapter, we'll unfurl the story of how aging twirls with our digestive system, and I'll share the secret recipe for keeping our internal garden blooming, even as the calendar pages keep turning.

As we step into the later chapters of our lives, it's not just our hair that decides to go gray or our skin that insists on telling the world our story through lines and creases. Our gut, that bustling metropolis within us, also faces its challenges. But fear not, my dear friends, for this is not a tale of woe. Instead, it's an invitation to a journey—a guide on nurturing our gut flora, ensuring it remains a thriving oasis of health, ready to face the golden glow of our later years with vim and vigor.

Stay tuned as I reveal how to keep the party in your gut lively, the conversations deep, and the atmosphere vibrant, no matter the number of candles on your birthday cake.

2.1 SAILING THROUGH THE SILVER YEARS: THE GUT'S VOYAGE THROUGH AGING

Physiological Changes

Let's spill the tea on what happens to our gut as we rack up those birthdays. It's like our gastrointestinal (GI) tract decides to take things down a notch, easing into a more leisurely pace. This means the process that shuffles food through our system, known as motility, starts to dawdle. Picture a once lively conveyor belt now preferring a leisurely stroll, which can make our bodies less efficient at dealing with the feasts we lay before it.

And it doesn't stop there. Our production line of stomach acid and digestive enzymes, crucial for breaking down our grub, also decides to slack off a bit. It's as though our digestive workforce has opted for early retirement, leaving us in the lurch, trying to wring every last nutrient from our meals.

Impact on Digestion

These changes can throw a major disruption in digestion. Slower motility means constipation could become your new, uninvited dinner guest more often than you'd like. And with our stomach acid and enzymes on a go-slow, we might feel bloated or overly full after meals, not to mention the hassle of getting enough nutrients. It's like trying to juice an orange with a pair of old, blunt scissors—frustrating and ineffective.

Common Gut-related Aging Issues

As we step gracefully into our senior years, a few familiar gut health nemeses might start to pop up:

- **Constipation**: Becomes more of a regular annoyance due to that leisurely gut motility.
- **Gastroesophageal reflux disease (GERD):** Might decide to join the party, as changes in the GI tract invite stomach acid to places it really shouldn't be.
- **Diverticular disease:** Those little pouches in the colon wall become more likely to form as nature's way of adding pockets to our internal wardrobe.
- **Peptic ulcers**: The risk increases, partly because of the long-term guest list of medications many of us accumulate over the years.

Adaptive Strategies

But here's the good news: the situation is far from dire. There are a variety of strategies to keep your gut humming along:

- **Stay Active:** Think of regular, gentle exercise as taking your digestive system out for a daily excursion. It keeps things moving and grooving.
- **Hydrate**: Keeping well-watered helps fend off constipation. Consider it the essential oil for your internal machinery.
- **Fiber Up:** Adding fiber-rich foods to your diet is like having a friendly internal broom sweeping through your digestive tract to keep it clean and tidy.
- **Mindful Eating:** Taking time to chew thoroughly and savor your meals enhances the dining experience and

ensures your body can soak up all the nutritional goodness.

- **Regular Check-ups**: Regular chats with your healthcare provider can help avoid potential gut grievances, ensuring they're nipped in the bud.

By weaving these habits into the tapestry of our daily lives, we can ensure our gut continues to serve us well as we age. Embracing the changes that come with aging, with a dash of humor and a spoonful of wisdom, allows us to maintain digestive health and our zest for life, ensuring we can savor every moment of our golden years with grace and gusto.

2.2 NAVIGATING TUMMY TROUBLES IN OUR TWILIGHT YEARS: A GUIDE FOR THE SAGE AND SAVVY

Ah, the golden years—a time when life should be as smooth as a well-aged whiskey, filled with leisure, laughter, and maybe a bit of mischief. Yet, it seems Mother Nature has a sense of humor, introducing a few digestive curveballs that can throw us off our game. But fear not! Identifying these pesky intruders is half the battle, paving the way for strategies that ensure our digestive system becomes a partner in crime, not a party pooper.

Common Culprits

As we gracefully ascend the age ladder, a few uninvited guests tend to make their presence known. Gastritis, that grumpy inflammation of the stomach lining, decides to crash the party, bringing along its dietary restrictions. Gallstones, those pesky pebbles of discomfort, can block the flow of digestive juices, leading to some rather un-ladylike expressions of pain. GERD, the unwelcome belcher, turns the simple joy of eating into a game of digestive roulette, while the specter of colorectal cancer nudges us towards being vigilant with our health checks.

Culinary Concoctions for Comfort

Our pantry and plate wield the power to tame these rebellious rebels.

- **Gastritis**: Sideline the spicy, acidic, or fried temptations in favor of gentler fare. Think of bananas, rice, and applesauce as your gut's best buddies, offering solace without the sass.
- **Gallstones:** A balanced diet that flirts with fiber and winks at healthy fats while giving the cold shoulder to high-cholesterol items can keep those stones at bay.
- **GERD**: Opt for smaller, more frequent meals over the belt-busting banquets, and steer clear of the culinary troublemakers like chocolate, caffeine, and alcohol. A little elevation of your sleeping quarters can also prevent those pesky acids from gatecrashing your esophagus.
- **Colorectal Cancer Prevention:** A diet that romances fruits, vegetables, and whole grains, coupled with a dalliance with regular exercise, can play hard to get with cancer risks.

When the Kitchen Isn't Enough

Despite our best culinary efforts, medical cavalry sometimes needs to be called in. Persistent gastritis may require acid-reducing champions or stomach-lining protectors. Severe gallstone symptoms could lead to a gallbladder eviction. GERD, stubborn as an old mule, might need antacids or proton pump inhibitors to keep it in check. Colorectal cancer, that thief in the night, is best thwarted by early detection through regular screenings.

A Holistic Waltz

Embracing a holistic waltz, where every step and turn considers the body's interconnected marvels, can boost the effectiveness of our efforts.

- **Exercise**: A gentle promenade, whether walking or tai chi, keeps the digestive orchestra in tune, reducing stress and encouraging a happy gut dance.
- **Stress Management:** Techniques like deep breathing, meditation, or indulging in hobbies knit a cozy blanket of calm, soothing our digestive woes.
- **Hydration:** A steady flow of fluids ensures our internal plumbing remains unclogged, combating constipation with the elegance of a flowing river.
- **Social Spice:** The zest of life comes from our connections. A robust support network can season our days joyfully, easing stress and its digestive discord.

Weaving these strategies into the fabric of our daily lives not only shores up our digestive health but polishes our golden years until they genuinely sparkle. So, here's to navigating the twilight years with wisdom, wit, and a well-behaved tummy, making every moment count.

2.3 THE ART OF EATING WELL: CRAFTING A MENU FOR THE MATURE PALETTE

Ah, the adventure of aging! It's like our bodies decide to rewrite the rulebook on what they need to thrive, particularly when dining at the table of life. As our metabolism chooses to take a leisurely stroll rather than a brisk jog, our digestive system becomes a tad more finicky about what it takes, and tailoring our diet becomes an essential craft. It's not just about filling the plate;

it's about painting a culinary masterpiece that caters to our evolved nutritional needs without skimping on the pleasure of a good meal.

Nutritional Tweaks for the Timeless Diner

As the years grace us with their presence, our bodies whisper (sometimes shout) for a change in the dietary script. Calories take a backseat, making room for nutrient-rich foods that punch above their weight. Spotlight on vitamins D and B12, calcium, and all-important fiber—our backstage heroes for bone health, brain function, and keeping the digestive dance smooth.

Embracing these nutritional shifts means getting friendly with foods that tickle our taste buds and fill our nutritional coffers. Imagine a palette bursting with fruits, vegetables, lean proteins, and grains that keep the body humming and the spirit soaring.

Superfoods: The VIP Guests at the Senior's Table

Certain foods have stolen the limelight, earning their stripes as 'superfoods' for their nutrient density and added boons for gut health and overall vim and vigor:

- **Blueberries:** Akin to nature's candy, brimming with antioxidants to keep inflammation at bay.
- **Nuts and Seeds:** The perfect ensemble of almonds, chia, and flaxseeds, blending fiber and healthy fats in a harmony that delights heart and mind.
- **Leafy Greens:** The green brigade of spinach, kale, and their kin marching in with an arsenal of vitamins and fiber.
- **Fatty Fish:** The swimmers—salmon, mackerel, sardines— dripping with omega-3 fatty acids to fight inflammation and keep our brains as sharp as our wit.

- **Whole Grains:** The steady energy suppliers like quinoa, barley, and oats keep our digestive narrative smooth and engaging.

Incorporating these stars into your daily dining doesn't need to be a Broadway production. Snack on nuts, blend a berry smoothie, toss up a green salad with a slice of fatty fish, and you've got a day's worth of nutrient-packed eating that's as delicious as it is wise.

When the Menu Needs a Boost: Supplements

Even the most well-crafted diet might have gaps, especially when the sun isn't enough for our vitamin D needs or when B12 decides to play hard to get. Here's where supplements might step in to take a bow. However, always consult with the director of your health care before adding any new act to your nutritional plan, ensuring the supplements complement your script without stepping on the toes of any medications you're already courting.

Meal Planning: The Director's Cut

Crafting meals that sing to our nutritional needs and delight our palates may seem daunting, but it's more about embracing the art of simplicity and variety:

- **Batch Cooking:** Think of it as preparing your TV dinners with a gourmet twist. Freeze portions for when the kitchen seems miles away.
- **Keep It Simple, Sweetheart:** Who said nutritious can't be delicious? Simple dishes that spotlight fresh, whole ingredients often carry the most flavor and health benefits.
- **Flavor's the Spice of Life:** With taste buds potentially taking a different stance in our golden years, herbs and spices become our best friends, adding zest and zeal to every bite.

- **Embrace the Rainbow:** Ensure your menu keeps boredom at bay by inviting a spectrum of foods to grace your table, each a star in its own right.
- **Hydration's Part of the Ensemble:** Soups, smoothies, and the humble glass of water play their roles in keeping us hydrated, supporting digestion, and adding to our nutrient intake.

By painting our plates with the vibrant colors of nutrient-dense foods, flirting with superfoods, judiciously using supplements, and curating our meals with creativity and care, we feed our bodies and nourish our souls. Here's to relishing every meal as a feast for the senses, ensuring that as we journey through our golden years, we do so with enthusiasm, grace, and a well-fed glow.

2.4 THE MAGIC WAND OF AGING: FIBER'S LEADING ROLE

As we waltz into the later acts of life's grand play, fiber steps onto the stage like a seasoned conductor, ready to orchestrate the symphony of our digestive system with grace and aplomb. This unsung hero of the dietary world deserves a standing ovation, especially from the silver-haired audience, for its virtuoso performance in keeping our internal rhythms flowing smoothly.

The Ins and Outs of Fiber

Fiber, darling, is essentially your gut's best friend—a dietary dynamo that keeps things moving with the elegance of a ballroom dance. It comes in two star-studded varieties: soluble, which plays the mysterious dissolver in water, creating a gel that eases digestion, and insoluble, the bold non-dissolver that adds volume to our performances (or bowel movements, to be precise). For us, the distinguished crowd, striking the right balance between these two is crucial to encore performances of regularity and a bouquet of health benefits, including heart health, blood sugar control, and maintaining a trim waistline by keeping hunger at bay.

Casting Fiber in Your Daily Diet

Incorporating fiber into our daily script is less about auditions and more about welcoming a cast of nutrient-rich foods into the fold:

- **Fruits:** Apples, berries, and oranges are not merely acts of nature's sweetness; they're fibrous understudies waiting in the wings.
- **Vegetables:** The likes of broccoli, carrots, and Brussels sprouts step into the spotlight, offering a satisfying crunch of fiber.
- **Legumes:** Scene-stealers like beans, lentils, and chickpeas bring depth to the plot with their hearty fiber content and protein punch.
- **Whole Grains**: Morning till night, oats, barley, and quinoa can play versatile roles, from the opening act of breakfast to the closing scene of dinner.
- **Nuts and Seeds:** Almonds and chia seeds make for a delightful intermission snack, sprinkling fiber across salads, yogurts, or oats.

Integrating these characters into your daily dining can be done without a director's cut. Simple acts like berry-topped cereal, a vibrant veggie lunch, or a nutty afternoon snack can elevate your fiber intake with minimal fuss.

The Art of Introducing Fiber

Ramping up your fiber intake is akin to rehearsing a new dance routine—start slow, let your body adjust to the latest moves, and gradually increase the tempo to avoid missteps like bloating or gas. A food diary can be your backstage pass, offering insights into how different foods play their parts and how your body responds to each scene.

Hydration: Fiber's Dance Partner

Remember to underestimate the power of hydration significantly when boosting your fiber intake. Think of water as the choreographer that ensures fiber's performance doesn't miss a beat, aiding in its mission to soften and smooth the way for regularity. Failing to hydrate appropriately can turn fiber's tale into a tragedy, so keep the water flowing. Maintaining this fluid harmony is crucial for a standing ovation, whether through the classic eight glasses a day, herbal teas, or water-laden fruits and veggies.

By embracing fiber as the lead in our dietary ensemble, we support a seamless digestive narrative and enhance our overall well-being. With a thoughtful approach to fiber's role and ensuring adequate hydration, we can ensure the show goes on, dazzling and delightful, into our golden years.

2.5 FRIENDLY BACTERIA AND THEIR FIBER FEAST: GUT HARMONY IN OUR ENCORE YEARS

In the grand opera of our gut, a lively cast of microorganisms takes center stage, playing a critical role in our health's unfolding drama, particularly as the spotlight dims on our younger years. This ensemble within us, known as the gut microbiota, experiences a shake-up as we step into the autumn of our lives, affecting our well-being in ways that are as fascinating as they are vital. Enter stage left: probiotics and prebiotics, our gut's most dependable understudies, ready to ensure the show goes smoothly as we embrace our senior years.

The Gut's Changing Seasons

As the pages of the calendar turn, the diversity in our gut's microbial community tends to wane, like a garden in winter. This shift leaves our inner ecosystem vulnerable, impacting everything from fending off invaders to processing the banquet of life. It's a time when the wisdom of probiotics and prebiotics become invaluable, helping to balance vitality and vigor.

Probiotics: The Gut's Benefactors

Think of probiotics as the gut's nurturing nannies, live microorganisms that tend to our digestive well-being, keeping harmful bacteria at bay and supporting our immune system's defenses. For those of us enjoying the wisdom that comes with age, probiotics offer a helping hand to counteract the natural decline in our gut's microbial variety. They're the reinforcements to ease gastrointestinal upsets, bolster our gut wall's defenses, and keep unwanted guests like infections in check.

Prebiotics: The Feast for Our Friends

While probiotics are the stars, prebiotics are the scriptwriters, providing the essential fibers that nourish our gut's beneficial bacteria. These non-digestible fibers act as a banquet for our microbial allies, fermenting in the gut to create a flourishing environment where probiotics can thrive. It's a partnership that enhances our digestive health, ensuring our nutrient absorption is top-notch, and our immune system remains spry and ready for action.

Casting Probiotics and Prebiotics in Your Daily Diet

Bringing these gut-friendly agents into your daily repertoire can be an enjoyable culinary exploration:

- **Probiotic Provisions**: Venture into the world of fermented delights. A dollop of live-culture yogurt on your breakfast, a glass of kefir, or a forkful of sauerkraut can introduce probiotics to your gut's cast. When choosing yogurt, peek at the label for a nod to live cultures, ensuring you get the real deal.
- **Prebiotic Picks**: Onions, garlic, bananas, and a parade of whole grains stand ready to enrich your dishes with prebiotic prowess. These ingredients script a flavorful meal and set the stage for a thriving gut microbiota.
- **Supplemental Stars:** If the idea of fermented foods doesn't raise your appetite, probiotic supplements can step into the role. The key is to consult your healthcare maestro to find the right strain and encore that harmonizes with your unique health script.
- **A Diverse Ensemble:** Variety isn't just the spice of life; it's the cornerstone of a thriving gut. Experimenting with different probiotic and prebiotic sources can make each meal an act of nourishment and discovery, ensuring your gut's microbial community remains as diverse and vibrant as a Broadway cast.

As we choreograph our diets to include these vital players, we're not just feeding ourselves; we're conducting an orchestra that plays the symphony of our health. In their supportive roles, probiotics and prebiotics help maintain the balance and richness of our gut flora, ensuring that as we advance in our years, our inner ecosystem remains a well-tuned ensemble capable of supporting our health and happiness. In this act of our lives, embracing the duo of probiotics and prebiotics is akin to ensuring the show goes on splendidly and without a hitch as we continue to explore and enjoy the richness of our encore years.

SUMMARY AND HOMEWORK FOR CHAPTER TWO

As we journey through the chapters of our lives, reaching the narrative rich with wisdom and grace that our later years bring, it's crucial to remember the role of our internal ecosystem – our gut health – in maintaining our vitality and zest for life. Chapter Two is a lovingly crafted guide to nurturing our gut flora, ensuring it remains a thriving oasis of health. Here, we unfold the secrets to keeping the gut's lively party going, ensuring deep conversations and a vibrant atmosphere, no matter how many candles light up our birthday cakes.

In our silver years, the digestive tract, like a well-loved book, shows signs of wear, its pages turning more slowly. But with a sprinkle of humor, a dash of wisdom, and a hearty dose of science-backed knowledge, we can write a story of digestive health that supports, rather than detracts from, the rich tapestry of our lives.

Action Plan for a Flourishing Gut:

- **Embrace Fermented Foods:** Dive into the world of yogurt, kefir, sauerkraut, and kimchi. Start small, enjoy the diversity, and listen to your body's cues. These foods are not just snacks but your gut's best allies.
- **Fiber is Your Friend:** Introduce more vegetables, fruits, legumes, and whole grains into your diet. Be creative, make your meals colorful and varied, and increase fiber intake gradually to keep your digestive system humming happily.
- **Stay Hydrated:** Water is the lifeblood of a healthy gut. Aim for eight glasses daily, but remember, soups and smoothies also count! Hydration keeps the fiber moving and your gut garden lush.

- **Get Moving:** Regular, gentle exercise isn't just for your muscles; it's for your gut too. A brisk walk, a gentle yoga session, or even dancing in your living room can stimulate digestion and keep things flowing smoothly.
- **Mindful Eating:** Slow down, chew thoroughly, and savor every bite. Not only does this make every meal a celebration, but it also aids digestion and nutrient absorption.
- **Regular Check-ups:** Stay in tune with your body. Regular visits to your healthcare provider can catch potential issues early and keep your gut in the best shape for the adventures ahead.
- **Educate and Experiment:** Stay curious about your gut health. Read up, talk to professionals, and be bold and try new foods or recipes that could benefit your gut.
- **Connect and Share:** Your journey to maintaining a vibrant gut is worth sharing. Connect with friends, family, or support groups to share tips, recipes, and stories. A shared journey is a journey halved in burden and doubled in joy.

As we turn the pages to the next chapter of our lives, let's do so with intention and care, nurturing our gut health with the same love and attention we give to a cherished garden. Remember, a thriving gut means a thriving life full of vitality, joy, and the wisdom that comes with our golden years. Let's embrace this journey with open arms, a keen mind, and a spirit ready for adventure.

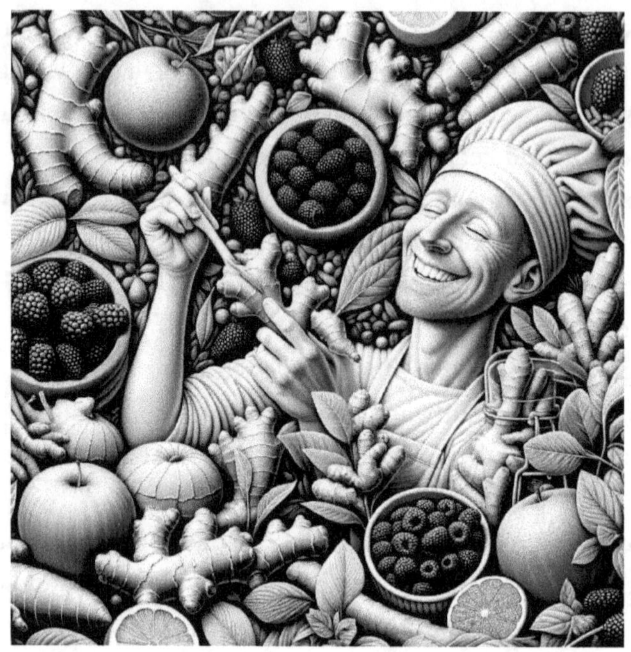

TENDING TO OUR INNER GARDEN: THE MAGIC OF FERMENTED FOODS

Step into your garden, and imagine it brimming with life, every leaf and petal flourishing because it's received the proper care. Your gut, my dear friends, is quite the same—a delicate garden within, teeming with life that thrives on the very best of what nature offers. Among the finest gifts we can bestow upon this inner ecosystem are the wonders of fermented foods. Just as a well-tended garden bursts with bounty, introducing these cultured delights into our diet is vital to nurturing a vibrant gut flora.

3.1 CULTURED CHARMS: FROM YOGURT TO THE WORLD BEYOND

The Probiotic Parade

Fermented foods are the unsung heroes of the digestive scene, loaded with probiotics that act as the gardeners of your gut, meticulously caring for its balance. These tiny allies are our internal landscapers, if you will, keeping the nasty bugs at bay, whipping up vital nutrients, and strengthening the walls of our digestive tract. Imagine them as your gut guardians, dedicated to your digestive harmony, bolstering your immunity, and possibly even brightening your mood.

The Fermented Family

While yogurt and kefir have long been the celebrities of the fermented food world, let's not forget about their equally impressive relatives:

- **Sauerkraut:** This tangy treasure isn't just for topping hot dogs; it's a probiotic powerhouse, ready to revitalize your gut garden.
- **Kimchi:** A fiery ferment from Korea, this veggie concoction brings both zest and zing to your plate and a crowd of friendly bacteria.
- **Tempeh:** A gift from Indonesia, this soy sensation offers a satisfying bite and a nutty nuance alongside a bevy of beneficial microbes.
- **Miso:** Hailing from Japan, this savory paste transforms soups and sauces with its deep umami, all while ferrying probiotics to your grateful gut.

Dabbling in these fermented delights introduces not just a medley of flavors but a mosaic of probiotics to your gut, each with its unique tune to play in the symphony of your health.

Weaving Them Into Your Wholesome Diet

Infusing your meals with these fermented wonders can be an adventure in taste and health. Here are a few pointers:

- **Begin Gently:** If you're new to the fermented scene, ease these foods into your diet to let your gut acquaint itself gracefully.

- **Mix and Match:** Toss some sauerkraut into your salads, whip kefir into your morning smoothies, dissolve miso into warming broths, or swap out the usual protein for tempeh at home in your next stir-fry.
- **DIY Delights:** Embark on the rewarding journey of fermenting at home with something simple like sauerkraut. A little cabbage, a pinch of salt, and patience can yield delicious, probiotic-rich rewards.

A Note of Caution:

Though generally beneficial, fermented foods can sometimes stir the pot for a few of us.

Moderation Matters: Diving too deep too quickly into fermented foods can lead to bloating or gas. Let your gut adapt at its own pace.

- **Sodium Watch:** Keep an eye on the salt, especially with ferments like sauerkraut and miso. Opt for low-sodium varieties if salt is a concern for you.
- **Histamine Heads-Up:** For those sensitive to histamine, fermented foods might prompt unwelcome reactions like headaches or digestive discomfort.

With a mindful approach to integrating these cultured treasures, you can tap into their myriad benefits, turning your dietary routine into a celebration of gut health and well-being.

Embracing the diversity and nourishment fermented foods offer is akin to planting a lush, varied garden within, ensuring our gut flora thrives in vibrant health. With each fermented bite, we indulge in nature's culinary artistry and fortify our internal garden, cultivating well-being that radiates from the inside out.

3.2 WEAVING MAGIC WITH FIBER: A CULINARY JOURNEY THROUGH THE SILVER YEARS

Venturing through the rich tapestry of our later years, fiber emerges as the unsung hero of our digestive saga, much like the fertile earth that cradles the roots of a blooming garden. This stalwart nutrient, often overshadowed by flashier dietary players, is, in fact, the backbone of our gut's well-being. It acts as the diligent groundskeeper of our digestive tract, sweeping away the debris and laying a feast for our gut's microscopic allies.

Fiber: The Gut's Best Friend

The role of fiber in our digestive health ensemble is multifaceted. Beyond its renowned ability to prevent the dreaded slow march of constipation, fiber is a linchpin in nurturing a harmonious gut microbiome. Unassumingly, as fiber passes through our system, it arrives in the colon not as waste but as a banquet for our beneficial bacteria. The resulting fermentation performance produces short-chain fatty acids—these little wonders nourish our colon cells, keep our immune system in tip-top shape, and dial down inflammation, showcasing the elegant dance between our dietary habits and the bustling life within our guts.

A Smorgasbord of Fiber

The culinary world is brimming with fibrous treasures, each bringing its unique flavor and zest to the table.

- **Vegetables**: From the hearty artichoke to the humble pea and the robust Brussels sprout, vegetables are not merely sides but stars laden with fiber.
- **Fruits**: Berries, pears, and apples, donned in their natural skins, offer a sweet path to ramping up our fiber intake.
- **Whole Grains:** The likes of farro, barley, and bran are the

unsung heroes, providing not just texture and substance
but a significant fiber boost.

These are but a few characters in the vast cast of fiber-rich foods
available to us, each capable of enriching our gut's ecosystem while
delighting our palates.

Fiber with Flair: Elevating the Everyday

Infusing our diet with fiber need not be a drab affair; it's an opportunity to embark on a culinary voyage that marries nutrition with
flavor.

- **Breakfast Brilliance:** Imagine kicking off the day with a
  fiber-filled breakfast burrito, where scrambled eggs meet
  black beans, avocado, and a splash of salsa, all snugly
  wrapped in a whole-grain tortilla.
- **Luncheon Luxe**: A midday quinoa salad tossed with an
  array of roasted veggies, offers a crunch that's as satisfying
  to the ear as it is to the gut.
- **Snack-time Symphony:** For those moments of
  peckishness, almond butter on apple slices or a hearty
  cracker topped with cottage cheese and cucumber can be a
  fiber-rich serenade.
- **Evening Elegance:** A dinner where baked salmon rests on
  a bed of farro, mingled with spinach and mushrooms,
  closes the day on a high note of fiber harmony.

These culinary creations showcase fiber's versatility, proving that a
diet rich in this essential nutrient can be as delectable as
nourishing.

Tailoring the Fiber Tapestry

While the chorus sings the praises of fiber, it's essential to remember that the melody must be adjusted to the individual. The quantity of fiber that serenades one's system to harmony might differ from person to person, influenced by the unique rhythms of our bodies and lives. Here's how to conduct your fiber intake with grace:

- **Gentle Beginnings:** For those tuning their systems to the fiber frequency, a gradual increase allows the gut to adapt without discord.
- **Hydration Harmony:** A chorus of fluids alongside fiber ensures the digestive concert plays out without a hitch.
- **Guidance from the Maestro:** Consulting with a healthcare professional provides a tailored score for managing fiber intake, ensuring the digestive symphony plays on beautifully.

In embracing fiber, we weave a narrative of digestive wellness that supports the vibrant ecosystem within our gut. By carefully incorporating fiber-rich foods into our diet, we create a melody that nurtures our gut microbiota, ensuring our digestive health remains robust and vibrant. This chapter is a testament to the power of fiber, inviting us to explore and enjoy the culinary journey toward optimal gut health underpinned by the natural magic of fiber.

3.3 QUENCHING THE INNER THIRST: WHY YOUR GUT LOVES A GOOD HYDRATION PLAN

Ah, water—nature's elixir, as plain as an old shoe but as vital as the air we breathe. In the grand scheme of things, especially in our golden encore, water plays the unsung hero in the opera of our digestive health. It's the backstage crew that ensures the show goes on, aiding digestion, keeping the pipes flowing, and ensuring our internal garden stays verdantly lush.

The Dance of Water and Digestion

Water and our digestive system share a tango that's as timeless as crucial. Imagine water as the gentle rain that revives a thirsty garden; it breathes life into our digestive tract, ensuring nutrients are embraced, and waste is shown the door with grace. It softens the stools for their grand exit, helping dodge the discomfort of constipation—a pesky interloper that no one wants at their tea party. And let's not forget water is the maestro for our digestive enzymes, orchestrating the breakdown of our meals into the symphony of nutrients our bodies dance to.

How Much is Enough?

The oft-quoted "eight glasses a day" is more of a guideline than a gospel. It's the curtain raiser for the individualized art of hydration.

Considerations such as the encore of physical activity, which calls for more water to replace what we've sweat out, and the climate of our environment play their parts. The stage of life we're in and our health's overall plot line also influence how much water we should sip to keep our inner workings humming harmoniously.

The Supporting Cast: Water-Rich Foods

Our plates can become oases of hydration when we invite water-rich foods to the party. Cucumbers and lettuce, those crunchy champions of hydration, delights, and juicy fruits like watermelon and strawberries, quench our thirst and serenade our taste buds with their flavors. These culinary delights offer a refreshing twist to our hydration efforts, ensuring our fluid intake is as delicious as beneficial.

Listening to Your Body's Cues

Understanding when our body is sending out an SOS for hydration is vital.

Thirst is the headliner, but there are understudies like dry mouth, fatigue, and a curtain call for more frequent bathroom breaks or noticing your urine taking on a darker hue. Should headaches or dizziness step onto the stage, it's high time to take a hydration intermission, rejuvenating our body's performance with a glass of water or a hydrating snack.

Incorporating a hydration strategy into the script of our daily lives elevates water from a mere supporting role to a star performer in our digestive health. It's a fluid foundation supporting complex processes and ensuring our digestive tract remains well-tuned. By tuning into our hydration needs, indulging in water-rich foods, and responding to our body's cues, we keep our gut garden in bloom, nourished by the life-affirming essence of water. So, here's to lifting a glass (of water, mind you) to our health, ensuring that every day is a hydrated journey towards well-being.

3.4 DOUSING THE FLAMES: A CULINARY FIRE BRIGADE FOR YOUR GUT

Now, let's talk about the fire within, and I don't mean the burning passion for a late-night tango. I'm referring to inflammation in the gut, a sneaky little blaze that can lead to all sorts of hullabaloos-like bloating and those more bothersome conditions we whisper about. The good news? We've got a fire extinguisher in the form of an anti-inflammatory diet, ready to calm those internal embers and bring back peace.

The Gut's Fiery Foe

Inflammation in our digestive theater can turn a harmonious performance into a bit of a drama, leading to a range of discomforts and potentially setting the stage for more severe health plot twists. Triggered by various culprits, including our diet, this inflammatory response is like an overly critical audience, causing disruption where there was once ease. However, as we choose our theater plays wisely, we can select foods that soothe rather than stoke the flames.

Nature's Anti-inflammatory Cast

In her wisdom, Mother Nature offers a pantry filled with ingredients known for their anti-inflammatory prowess. Let's shine a spotlight on a few stars:

- **Turmeric:** A spice that's not just for making your curry vibrant but is packed with curcumin, known for putting out inflammatory fires. A dash here and there in your cooking, and you're already on your way to calming the flames.
- **Ginger:** This root is like the cool aunt who knows just how to soothe your woes. Brewed in tea or grated into

your stir-fry, it's a versatile performer in the anti-inflammatory show.

- **Berries:** These little jewels—strawberries, blueberries, raspberries—are delicious and come loaded with antioxidants, ready to battle inflammation one bite at a time.
- **Leafy Greens:** The robust supporting cast of spinach, kale, and chard, rich in antioxidants, are the understudies that deserve a standing ovation for their anti-inflammatory effects.

Incorporating these foods into your daily diet script can be simpler than memorizing Shakespeare, focusing on adding a sprinkle of this and a handful of that to shift the scene towards anti-inflammatory eating gradually.

Scripting Your Anti-inflammatory Diet

Turning the spotlight towards anti-inflammatory foods can start with easy yet flavorful script revisions:

- **Spice It Up:** Introduce turmeric and ginger into your culinary repertoire. They're like seasoned actors who know how to improve a scene.
- **Berry Good Snacks:** Swap those processed nibbles for a handful of berries. After all, they're nature's candy with a side of health benefits.
- **Embrace the Greens:** Include a leafy green at every curtain call, be it as a salad star, a sautéed sidekick, or a smoothie extra.

Small steps, yes, but each one is a stride towards reducing the internal inferno, setting the stage for a more peaceful bodily domain.

The Long Run

Adopting an anti-inflammatory diet is akin to investing in a season ticket for a healthier life. The benefits extend far beyond quieting the gut's grumbles, potentially playing a role in

- **Gut Harmony:** Reducing inflammation helps keep the integrity of your gut's lining in check, making for a happier digestive narrative.
- **Boosted Immunity:** A balanced gut microbiome is like having your own personal bodyguard, ready to defend against unwanted invaders.
- **Chronic Disease Prevention:** Keeping inflammation at bay is like avoiding the drama of chronic conditions, including heart disease and diabetes.

Embarking on an anti-inflammatory diet is a journey of culinary discovery, finding which foods bring comfort and joy while soothing the gut. It's about tuning into your body's needs and answering with thoughtful nourishment, choosing dishes that tickle the taste buds and contribute to a harmonious, healthy life. Here's to making each meal a step towards extinguishing the flames of inflammation, paving the way for a serene, flourishing existence.

3.5 TAMING TUMMY TROUBLES WITH THE FODMAP STRATEGY

Wandering through the maze of digestive wellness, we stumble upon a beacon of hope for those of us battling the bloat and other unsavory belly woes: the FODMAP diet. This isn't your run-of-the-mill diet fad but a science-backed approach showing promise for folks wrestling with digestive discomfort, especially the brave souls navigating the choppy waters of Irritable Bowel Syndrome (IBS).

Decoding FODMAPs

FODMAP—an acronym that sounds like it belongs in a spy novel—stands for Fermentable Oligosaccharides, Disaccharides, Monosaccharides, And Polyols. Simply put, they're a bunch of carbohydrates that can cause a ruckus in the small intestine because they're tough to digest. When they stroll undigested into the large intestine, they become a feast for gut bacteria, leading to gas and water being drawn into the gut and, subsequently, a party of bloating, cramps, and discomfort. High-FODMAP culprits include some fruits like apples and pears, dairy delights rich in lactose, wheaty wonders, and certain sweeteners that sound more like space-age polymers.

The Low-FODMAP Lifeline

Embracing a low-FODMAP diet is akin to donning a superhero cape for your gut. It significantly dials down the internal drama by curtailing the intake of fermentable mischief-makers, aiming to reduce the symptoms for individuals with IBS. Picture it as clearing the stage of overzealous actors so the gut can perform its soliloquy in peace. Research tips its hat to this dietary approach, showing many with IBS can take a bow, enjoying a reduction in their gastrointestinal encore.

Charting the Low-FODMAP Voyage

Embarking on the low-FODMAP journey unfolds in two acts: the elimination and the grand reintroduction.

- **Elimination:** This opening act involves giving high-FODMAP foods the cold shoulder for about 3-6 weeks to quiet the gut's uproarious applause.

- **Reintroduction:** With symptoms hopefully taking a curtain call, high-FODMAP foods are slowly invited back, one at a time, to pinpoint which ones deserve a starring role in causing discomfort. It's a culinary detective story, identifying the culprits behind the scenes.

While it might seem like a plot twist in your dining narrative, many find this structured approach a guiding light to uncovering their personal food sensitivities.

Personalizing Your Script

The low-FODMAP diet isn't a one-size-fits-all affair. Our gut microbiomes are as unique as our fingerprints, so what triggers a standing ovation in symptoms for one might not for another. The diet's finale should see you orchestrating a personalized menu that keeps the peace in your belly, allowing for the broadest range of foods without setting off any digestive alarms.

Navigating this with a dietitian experienced in the low-FODMAP blues can be like having a backstage pass. They help identify the high-FODMAP ensemble, suggest understudies, and ensure your nutritional needs are met without missing a beat.

Embarking on the low-FODMAP diet is akin to tuning your body's instrument to play the sweetest symphony. By carefully maneuvering through its phases, one can compose a diet that alleviates discomfort and brings into focus the harmonious interplay between diet and digestion. It's about crafting a culinary repertoire that supports your gut's well-being, allowing you to waltz through life with a happy belly. Through this dietary journey, we seek relief and gain a deeper understanding of our body's unique rhythms and needs, setting the stage for a vibrant, gut-happy existence.

SUMMARY, AND HOMEWORK FOR CHAPTER THREE

As we journey through the enchanting chapters of "Tending to Our Inner Garden," we've unearthed the quintessential elements for nurturing our gut's flora to full bloom. This guide has been your companion through the lush fields of fermented foods, the rich soil of fiber, the refreshing streams of hydration, the calming shades of anti-inflammatory foods, and the navigated paths of the FODMAP approach. Here's a lovingly crafted action plan to turn these insights into daily habits, ensuring your inner garden flourishes with vitality and joy.

Action Plan for Cultivating Your Inner Garden

Embrace the Cultured Charms:

- Start your day with a dollop of yogurt or kefir, blending it into your morning smoothie or enjoying it as is.
- Experiment by incorporating sauerkraut or kimchi into your lunches or dinners for that extra zing and gut health boost.
- Consider homemade fermentation projects like pickling vegetables – a delightful way to introduce beneficial bacteria into your diet.

Weave Magic with Fiber:

- Aim to incorporate a serving of fiber-rich foods into each meal, whether through a handful of berries for breakfast, a leafy green salad for lunch, or a side of quinoa for dinner.
- Snack on fiber-filled treats like nuts and seeds or fresh fruits and vegetables to keep your digestive system moving smoothly.

Quench Your Inner Thirst:

- Set a daily water intake goal that reflects your body's needs, considering activity level, climate, and personal health.
- Infuse your water with slices of cucumber, lemon, or berries for a refreshing twist that entices you to drink more throughout the day.
- Include water-rich foods like cucumbers, tomatoes, and watermelon to help meet your hydration needs.

Douse the Flames with Anti-inflammatory Foods:

- Incorporate turmeric and ginger into your cooking for their anti-inflammatory properties – they're perfect in teas, soups, and smoothies.
- Thanks to their potent anti-inflammatory effects, berries, leafy greens, and fatty fish are regular stars on your plate.
- Keep a food diary to identify foods that trigger inflammation and adjust your diet accordingly.

Navigate the FODMAP Terrain:

- If you suspect certain foods may be causing you digestive distress, consider trying a low-FODMAP diet under the guidance of a healthcare professional.
- Gradually eliminate high-FODMAP foods to identify triggers, then slowly reintroduce them to pinpoint which foods or ingredients you should avoid.
- Tailor your diet based on your discoveries, focusing on low-FODMAP foods you tolerate well to maintain variety and nutritional balance in your meals.

Cultivating Your Garden with Care

As you embark on this journey to tend to your inner garden, remember that patience, mindfulness, and a dash of curiosity are your best tools. Adjust your dietary habits gradually, listen attentively to your body's responses, and don't hesitate to seek guidance from nutrition experts, especially when navigating more complex strategies like the low-FODMAP diet.

By embracing these principles, you're not just feeding your body but nurturing your soul, ensuring that your internal ecosystem thrives. Let every meal be a step towards a more vibrant, balanced life, where digestive health is the cornerstone of your well-being. Here's to a flourishing garden within, where peace, vitality, and joy grow in abundance.

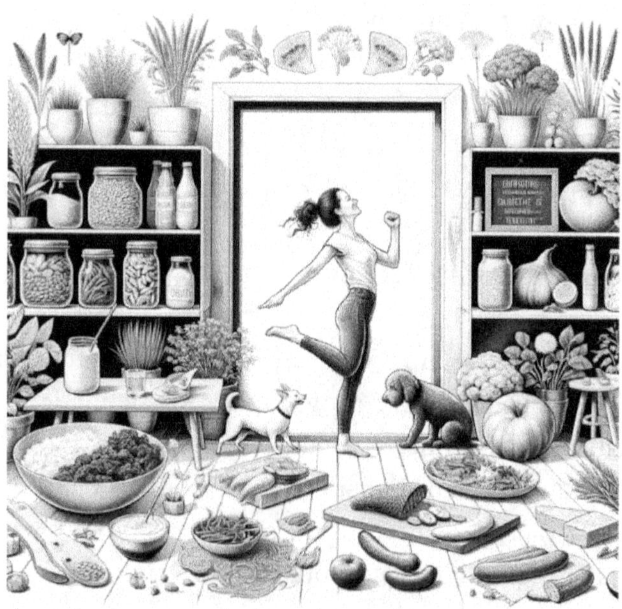

STEPPING AROUND DIGESTIVE LANDMINES: A GUIDE TO THE CULINARY CAUTION ZONE

Picture yourself meandering through a bustling bazaar, eyes wide at the cornucopia of culinary delights unfolding before you. From the sizzle of spicy delicacies to the allure of creamy confections, it's a veritable treasure trove of gustatory temptations. Yet, akin to navigating a crowded room in the dark, only some dishes are your friend regarding digestive peace. Knowing which foods to cozy up to and which to give the polite cold shoulder can be the secret to keeping your inner harmony in tune.

4.1 THE USUAL SUSPECTS: CULINARY CULPRITS BEHIND DIGESTIVE MISCHIEF

Much like a mystery novel, our dietary choices have their villains, often cloaked in delicious disguise, ready to wreak havoc on our unsuspecting digestive tract. Identifying these gastronomic gremlins is the first step in maintaining digestive contentment.

The Culinary Villains

- **Rich and Greasy Fare:** These high-fat foods can be likened to a traffic jam in your digestive highway, leaving you feeling like a stuffed suitcase and possibly fanning the flames of GERD.
- **Spicy Delicacies:** While they add zest to life, spicy foods can sometimes be too hot to handle for our digestive lining, inviting heartburn or discomfort to the party.
- **Leguminous Lecturers**: Beans and lentils, with all their fibrous wisdom, can also bring along gas and bloating, courtesy of their raffinose content.

Personal Culinary Maps

Our digestive landscapes are as varied as the plots of our lives, with certain foods playing the friend in one scene and the foe in another. It's essential to tune into your body's signals—what causes one person's digestive drama may be another's comfort food.

The Diary Detective

Maintaining a food diary is akin to playing detective in your digestive whodunit. Documenting your culinary adventures and the subsequent bodily responses can illuminate patterns, helping to identify which foods deserve a starring role and which are best kept in the background.

The Elimination Strategy

Embarking on an elimination diet is like thoroughly investigating your digestive grievances. By systematically removing and reintroducing suspects, you can pinpoint the precise actors responsible for any digestive discord, customizing your dietary script to suit your unique narrative.

Strategies for Skirting Sensitivities

Once you've spotlighted the foods stirring up internal unrest, there are tactics to mitigate their impact:

- **Portion Proportioning**: Sometimes, the villain is not the food but the sheer volume. Moderating portions can help keep the digestive peace.
- **Culinary Alchemy:** Transforming how you prepare foods can turn a digestive foe into a friend. For example, opting for steaming over frying might do the trick.
- **The Substitution Solution:** If certain edibles consistently play the antagonist, scouting for understudies can be a game-changer. Dairy dissenters, for instance, might find harmony in the plant-based alternatives.

Treading through the dietary landscape with a discerning eye doesn't mean sacrificing the joy of eating. With a sprinkle of wisdom and a dash of curiosity, you can craft a menu that sings harmoniously with your digestive system. Awareness, experimentation, and a touch of culinary creativity can turn the potential minefield of food sensitivities into a delightful garden path, leading to digestive well-being and a zestful life.

4.2 SWEET DILEMMA: NAVIGATING SUGAR'S STICKY WEB

Oh, sugar, you sly fox, you've danced into our lives with your sweet whispers, convincing us you're the sprinkle on our doughnuts, the fizz in our celebrations. Yet, behind your crystalline sparkle, you've been plotting a bit of digestive rebellion, haven't you? Let's pull back the curtain on this sweet charade and see how you've been stirring the pot in our gut health.

Sugar and Its Bittersweet Impact

Excess sugar, my dear friends, isn't just a matter of expanding waistlines; it's like throwing a lavish party in our gut where only the rowdy bacteria are invited, leaving our beneficial microbes sulking in the corner. This imbalance can lead to inflammation, like having too many unruly guests trampling through your garden, disrupting the harmony, and making a mess of the place. This inflammation isn't just about discomfort; it's laying down the welcome mat for more severe gate crashers like insulin resistance and some rather unwelcome autoimmune conditions.

In its cunning, the "Art of Sugar Disguise Sugar" has donned many a disguise, sneaking into our diets with the stealth of a cat burglar. It's not just the apparent sweets and sodas lurking in places you'd least suspect, from your morning toast to that "healthy" salad dressing. These hidden sugars are the masqueraders, with aliases ranging from the sophisticated "sucrose" to the more mundane "corn syrup." Becoming a label detective is our first line of defense, peering through our spectacles to uncover sugar's many pseudonyms and making choices that keep our inner garden in bloom.

Sweet Substitutions

Fear not, for the tale doesn't end in a sugary quagmire. In her wisdom, nature has provided a bounty of alternatives to keep our lives sweet without inviting chaos into our digestive system:

- **Fruits and Berries:** Ah, the natural confectioneries! Strawberries, apples, and their juicy kin offer a sweetness that comes with a fiber bonus, keeping our gut microbes doing the happy dance.
- **Stevia and Monk Fruit:** These are the modern magicians offering the sweet without the sour, so to speak, allowing us to indulge without upsetting the microbial balance.

- **Honey and Maple Syrup**: While they still wear the sugar cloak, they do so with a touch of elegance, bringing antioxidants and minerals to the party in moderation.

The Path to Less Sugar

Reducing sugar is akin to learning a new dance—one step at a time. Here's how we can glide gracefully away from sugar's grasp:

- **Ease Into It:** Cutting sugar cold turkey can lead to a tango with withdrawal symptoms. A slow waltz of reduction keeps the cravings and headaches at bay.
- **Whole Foods Waltz:** Embrace the ballroom of whole foods—vegetables, fruits, lean meats, and grains. They're the partners who won't step on your toes.
- **Smart Swaps:** Exchange that candy bar for a slice of dark chocolate and almonds. It's about choosing the dance partners who treat you right.
- **Hydration Harmony:** Swap the sugary symphony of sodas for the unmistakable melody of water, or perhaps an herbal tea ensemble for a refreshingly straightforward tune.

Adopting these steps invites a life where sugar no longer leads the dance, allowing us to twirl through our days with digestive harmony and a sweetness that doesn't turn sour.

CHAPTER 4.3 DAIRY DEBATE: THE CREAMY CONUNDRUM

Dairy, the once uncontested champion of breakfast tables and school lunches, now finds itself on trial in the court of public digestion. For some, it's akin to a loyal friend, comforting and always welcome. For others, it's more of a frenemy, with every encounter potentially leading to a tummy tumult. Let's meander through the dairy dilemma, shall we?

Lactose: The Mischief Maker

At the crux of this creamy quandary is lactose intolerance, a bit like being invited to a party only to discover you're not quite in tune with the host. When the body plays scrooge in lactase, the enzyme needed to digest lactose, dairy consumption can become a less-than-pleasant experience. Symptoms can range from bloating to a sprint to the nearest restroom. Then there's dairy sensitivity, a broader term encompassing reactions to dairy proteins such as casein and whey, further complicating our relationship with dairy.

Navigating Dairy-Free Waters

Fear not, for the world has blossomed with alternatives that mock dairy's essence with plant-based prowess:

- **Plant Milks:** From the nutty whispers of almond milk to the creamy caress of coconut milk, these alternatives frolic in your coffee and cereal without a hint of dairy drama.
- **Cheese, Please:** With the innovation of cashew spreads and coconut oil creations, dairy-free cheese has moved from fantasy to reality, ensuring pizzas and cheese boards remain in the repertoire.
- **Cool Treats:** Soy and almond have taken the plunge into yogurts and ice creams, ensuring dessert remains a sweet finale without the dairy downer.
- **Butter Substitutes:** Cooking and baking need to maintain their luster, with plant-based butters sliding smoothly onto the scene.

These dairy doppelgängers not only cater to those avoiding lactose but open a culinary treasure chest for the health-conscious and ethically inclined.

The Calcium and Vitamin D Duet

Ah, but what of calcium and vitamin D, those bastions of bone health, you ask? The plot thickens, but fear not:

- **Leafy Greens:** A hidden trove of calcium, these green marvels—kale, collard greens, and their leafy kin—stand ready to fortify.
- **Fortified Frontiers:** Plant milks and cereals, now donning armor of calcium and vitamin D, serve as worthy allies in the nutrient quest.
- **Bony Fish:** Sardines and salmon, with their calcium-rich skeletons, offer a hearty salute to bone health.
- **Nuts and Seeds:** A sprinkle of almonds or sesame seeds can add a crunchy dose of calcium to any dish.

And let's not forget, a spot of sunshine can do wonders for your vitamin D levels, though supplements are a trusty backup for the sun-shy.

To Dairy or Not to Dairy?

Ultimately, the dairy debate boils down to personal and bodily tales. It's a decision based on individual health, ethical leanings, and environmental considerations.

- **Experiment:** Dabble in dairy and dairy-free realms to discover what makes your gut sing.
- **Professional Wisdom:** A chat with a dietitian can illuminate the path, tailoring your dairy dalliance to your body's script.

- **Values:** For those walking the dairy-free path for ethical or environmental reasons, the journey is rich with community and resources.

Embracing or eschewing dairy is not about taking sides but finding the harmony that suits your body's chorus and your heart's song. Whether you toast with a glass of milk or a dairy-free alternative, the key is savoring the choice that brings you health, happiness, and a contented belly.

4.4 PROCESSED PITFALLS: DODGING THE CONVENIENCE TRAP

In this whirlwind era where everyone seems to be sprinting from task to task, processed foods have slyly nudged into our kitchens, whispering sweet nothings of convenience and time saved. Yet, what they don't advertise so loudly is their knack for throwing a spanner in the works of our digestive harmony. With a cocktail of additives, preservatives, and ingredients that sound more like entries in a science fair, these processed interlopers can make our gut flora throw up their tiny microbial hands in despair.

The Hidden Thorns of Processed Foods

Venturing down the aisles of processed temptations is like inviting foxes into the henhouse. Additives and preservatives, though marvelous for shelf life and taste, often play the villains, upsetting the delicate balance of our gut's ecosystem. This disruption can lead to the infamous "leaky gut," where unwanted substances make a break for the bloodstream, inciting inflammation and a host of uncomfortable encores. The high doses of sugar and salt often found masquerading in these foods contribute to the inflammatory fanfare, setting the stage for a less-than-joyful digestive drama.

Becoming a Label Linguist

Unraveling the mysteries of food labels is akin to decoding an ancient script. With a bit of know-how, you can become an adept translator:

- **Front vs. Back:** The front of the package is the food's pickup line, designed to charm. True intentions, however, are revealed in the ingredient list, and nutrition facts are on the back.
- **The List Tells All:** Ingredients parade in order of abundance. Eyebrow-raising additives or sugars leading the pack? Perhaps best left on the shelf.
- **Sugar's Many Masks:** Sugar, the master of disguises, appears under numerous aliases. Familiarize yourself with its various monikers to avoid unintentional indulgence. Fiber's Footprint: Many processed products are stripped of natural armor and fiber. Seek items where fiber is present and celebrated near the top of the list.

Embracing the Whole Food Waltz

Turning our backs on processed conveniences opens up a banquet of whole food wonders, each bursting with flavors untainted by artificial meddling:

- **Crunchy Swap:** Trade those bagged chips for nature's crunch - think slices of cucumber or bell peppers with a side of hummus or guacamole.
- **Grains in Their Prime:** Whole grains like quinoa, barley, or brown rice bring depth and nutrients to your plate, overshadowing their refined counterparts.
- **Nature's Candy:** Satisfy your sweet tooth with fruits'

natural goodness, offering a symphony of sweetness, fiber, and vitamins, unlike the empty serenade of sugary snacks.

Meal Prep: The Strategy for the Busy Bee

The prospect of daily culinary exploits from scratch may seem daunting, but with a sprinkle of planning and a dash of creativity, meal prep becomes less chore and more charm:

- **Batch Beauty:** A single cooking session can yield a week's worth of meals. Think big pots of soup, stews, or trays of roasted veggies, all customizable with a simple change of herbs or a new side.
- **Container Chic:** Quality containers are your allies, keeping your culinary creations fresh and making grab-and-go a breeze.
- **A Plan in Hand:** A weekly meal plan acts as your culinary compass, guiding your shopping list and ensuring every purchase has a purpose, cutting waste and stress.
- **Keep It Simple:** Not every meal needs to be a Michelin-star affair. Simple, wholesome dishes often pack the most punch in both nutrition and satisfaction.

Embracing a shift towards whole, unprocessed foods isn't just a boon for your gut; it's a love letter to your overall well-being. With a touch of foresight and a pinch of creativity, the world of whole foods unfolds like a treasure map, leading to vibrant health without falling prey to the siren song of processed convenience.

4.5 NIGHTSHADE NUANCES: A PEEK INTO POTATOES, TOMATOES, AND THEIR KIN

Oh yes, the nightshade family – a veritable masquerade ball of vegetables where tomatoes, potatoes, and peppers don their colorful capes, dancing through our diets with a mix of mystery and flair. While jazzing up our plates with a burst of color and flavor, these culinary staples come with a little-known twist for some: they can be the secret culprits behind a curtain of discomfort and inflammation for those sensitive to their particular brand of plant chemistry.

Nightshades, or the Solanaceae family if you're feeling botanical, are an eclectic troupe including not just the edible darlings we know and love but also some less savory characters (looking at you, belladonna). The common thread among them? Alkaloids are nature's pest control, which, while marvelous for the plants, can sometimes play havoc with certain human constitutions, leading to inflammation and exacerbating conditions like arthritis or causing a tummy ruckus.

Discovering whether you're in the audience affected by nightshades requires a bit of detective work:

- **Observation is Key:** Keep an eagle eye on how you feel after indulging in these veggie virtuosos. Any encore of discomfort or pain? Take note.
- **The Elimination Tango:** Consider taking a break from nightshades for a spell (a few weeks should do) to see if your symptoms take a bow and exit stage left.
- **The Solo Performance:** Bring them back into your diet one at a time, spotlighting each vegetable to see who might be the piece's villain.

Should you find yourself needing to steer clear of nightshades, there's no need to don a mourning veil for your culinary repertoire. The world of vegetables is vast and varied, ripe with understudies eager to take center stage:

- **Root Veggie Revue:** Swap in sweet potatoes or beets for a dose of comfort without the nightshade drama.
- **Leafy Green Ovations:** Spinach, kale, and their leafy companions bring a nutrient-rich vibrance to your plate.
- **Squash Spotlight:** From butternut to zucchini, squashes play well in any dish, from the hearty to the delicately spiced.
- **Herbal Harmonies:** Freshen your dishes with a chorus of herbs and spices. Basil, cilantro, and turmeric can sing the complex flavors you might miss; no nightshades are required.

Embarking on a culinary journey sans nightshades is not about restriction but exploration – an invitation to discover new flavors and textures that delight the palate and nurture the body. It's a testament to the richness of the food world, where every dietary twist opens the door to new culinary adventures.

In the grand scheme of our nutritional choices, understanding our body's unique responses to foods like nightshades underscores the personal nature of nutrition. It's a dance of discovery, where each step informs our path to well-being, reminding us that the best diet is tailored to our needs and stories. As we continue to navigate the culinary landscape, let's do so with curiosity, joy, and a sprinkle of creativity, crafting meals that resonate with our bodies and spirits.

SUMMARY AND HOMEWORK FOR CHAPTER FOUR

As we journeyed through the culinary caution zone in Chapter 4, we've uncovered the myriad ways our dietary choices can foster or foil our digestive health. From the high seas of processed foods to the murky waters of sugar's sweet embrace, navigating our way requires wisdom and wit. Here's a compass to guide you through the dietary dilemmas and help you maintain a symphony of digestive harmony:

- **Identify the Culprits**: Start by recognizing which foods tend to disrupt your digestive peace. Awareness is your first step, whether it's the decadent indulgence of high-fat foods, the fiery kick of spices, or the hidden sugars lurking in processed goods.
- **Become a Label Sleuth**: Equip yourself with the knowledge to decode food labels. This means looking beyond the marketing jargon to the nitty-gritty of ingredient lists, where sugars disguise themselves and additives hide.
- **Embrace Whole Foods:** Shift your culinary sails towards whole, unprocessed foods. These are the true treasures, rich in nutrients and devoid of the additives that often trigger digestive distress.
- **Experiment with Elimination**: Consider an elimination diet if certain foods consistently cast a shadow over your digestive well-being. This methodical approach can help you pinpoint specific sensitivities and tailor your diet to avoid these triggers.
- **Find Joyful Substitutes:** Discovering food sensitivities doesn't mean the end of culinary pleasure. Explore the vast array of substitutes available, from dairy-free delights to whole-grain wonders, and find new favorites that agree with your gut.
- **Listen to Your Body:** Consider how different foods affect you. Keep a food diary, note any symptoms, and adjust your diet accordingly. This personalized approach ensures your diet supports your digestive health and overall well-being.

- **Consult the Experts**: Don't navigate these waters alone. A dietitian or healthcare provider can offer tailored advice, helping you make informed choices that align with your health goals and dietary needs.
- **Savor the Journey:** Remember, exploring your dietary preferences and needs is not just about avoidance but discovery. Each step is an opportunity to learn more about what nourishes you, body and soul.

By arming yourself with knowledge and approaching your diet with curiosity and care, you can gracefully dance through the culinary caution zone. Embrace the adventure, and let your dietary choices be a harmonious reflection of your journey towards health and happiness

YOUR REVIEW COULD BE A GAME-CHANGER!

Share the Magic of Gut Instincts

"Kindness is the language which the deaf can hear, and the blind can see."

— MARK TWAIN

Did you know? People who share their blessings without expecting anything in return tend to live more joyful, fulfilling lives. So, why not sprinkle a little of that magic around, especially if it's as easy as sharing your thoughts?

I've got a small favor to ask...

Would you be willing to brighten someone's day, someone you've never even met, without seeking any glory for yourself?

Who might this person be, you wonder? Well, they're a bit like you. Maybe how you were before you knew the secrets of the gut-mind connection. Eager to learn, hoping to make a difference in their own life, but unsure where to start.

Our goal is to spread the word about the marvels of the mind-gut connection to everyone. Our entire endeavor is built around this mission. But we can only reach that lofty goal with your help.

Here's the deal: reviews matter. A lot. They can sway decisions, shape opinions, and most importantly, guide the curious and the seekers to their next great discovery. So, on behalf of a future gut-mind wizard you've yet to meet, I'm asking:

Would you kindly leave a review for this book?

This act of kindness doesn't cost a dime and takes less than a minute, yet it could profoundly impact another soul's journey. Your review might just be the nudge...

...another seeker needs to start their journey.

...a curious mind requires to dive deeper.

...a hopeful heart longs for to make that life-changing decision.

...an aspiring guru craves to share their newfound wisdom.

Are you feeling that warm, fuzzy glow yet? Here's how to make it happen—leave a review. It's quick, I promise!

Just use this QR code to share your thoughts:

https://shorturl.at/V77jy

If the idea of helping an unseen friend warms your heart, then you're definitely my kind of person. Welcome to the family!

I can't wait to guide you to unlock more secrets of your gut instincts in ways you never imagined. The insights waiting for you in the pages ahead will be transformative.

Thank you from the depths of my gut (and heart!). Let's dive back into the adventure.

With heartfeld gratitude,
~Your Guide on the Mind-Gut Journey~
Cherish Dutro

P.S. - Remember, sharing wisdom is the best kind of giving. If this book has touched your life, consider passing it on to someone else who might benefit. Let's spread the good vibes together!

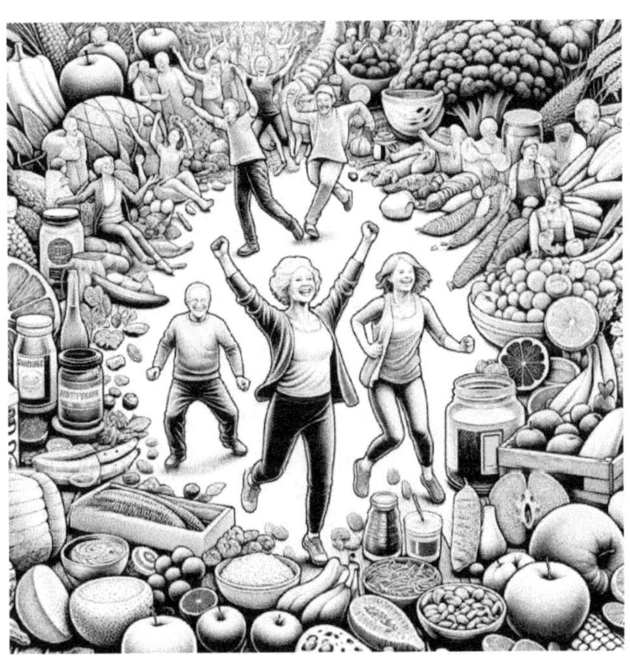

NAVIGATING LIFE'S STORMS WITH GRACE: STRESS AND OUR BELLY'S WHISPERS

Picture this: You're cozied up in your favorite nook, surrounded by the comforting silence that only the early hours can weave. Suddenly, the tranquility is shattered by the clang and clash of an unexpected storm—papers fluttering, knick-knacks rattling, and your serene bubble bursts. This little scenario, my dears, isn't too far off from what transpires in the delicate world of our gut when stress decides to crash our party. Just as our quiet nook couldn't keep calm, our digestive system struggled to keep its rhythm under the relentless stress dance. Stress, that unwelcome guest who doesn't know when to leave, doesn't just fray our nerves but also loves to tango with our gut.

5.1 THE INTRICATE WALTZ BETWEEN STRESS AND THE GUT: FINDING HARMONY

It's a Two-Way Convo

The tete-a-tete between stress and our gut is quite a sophisticated dialogue, each influencing the other profoundly. Stress, especially the kind that digs in its heels for the long haul, can usher in a host of tummy troubles—from mild discomforts to more persistent guests like Irritable Bowel Syndrome (IBS). It's quite the marvel (and a bit of a nuisance) how our gut, often dubbed our "second brain" due to its extensive neural network, picks up on our emotional upheavals. Stress has a knack for tossing a wrench in our digestive works, altering gut motility, and inviting symptoms such as bloating and an unpredictable schedule of bathroom visits.

Conversely, when our gut feels out of sorts, it sends distress signals up to the brain, potentially turning up the volume of stress and anxiety. Left to their own devices, stress and gut distress can spiral into a relentless loop, with each feeding into and amplifying the other.

The Long Stay of Chronic Stress

Chronic stress doesn't just pop by; it sets up residence, altering the rhythm of our gut and making the stomach lining more like a sieve —letting things through that ought to stay put. This can kickstart inflammation locally and body-wide, setting the stage for various health challenges beyond the digestive scene.

Harmonizing with Stress Management

To break free from this cycle, embracing stress management practices is key. Here are a handful of strategies to keep in your toolkit:

- **Embrace Movement:** Regular physical activity, from a spirited stroll to dancing in your living room, can dial down stress hormones and lift your spirits.
- **Breathe with Intention:** Practices like diaphragmatic breathing can be akin to sending a peace treaty to your nervous system, easing the tension that stress-induced digestive woes bring.

- **Seek Solace in Green Spaces**: Allowing yourself moments under the canopy of nature, be it a leisurely walk in the park or simply basking in your garden, can help soften the edges of stress.
- **Mind Your Stimulants**: Reducing caffeine and sugar can help lower the curtain on stress and its entourage, offering your gut some respite.

Real-Life Musings

Let's dip our spoons into the stew of life and fish out some real gems of wisdom, shall we? Picture a teacher navigating the choppy waters of education who finds an anchor in the calm seas of yoga and mindfulness. Not only did she manage to withstand the stormy waves of stress, but she also calmed the mutinous rumblings of her gut. Then there's the tale of a veteran who swapped his boots for gardening gloves, finding peace not in the silence of the battlefield but in the chatter of leaves and the earthy embrace of gardening. These ventures into the tranquil harbors of stress management soothed their spirits and brought harmony to their digestive tracts.

These narratives are more than just stories; they're lighthouses guiding us toward the shores of better health. They show us that by folding stress management into the fabric of our daily lives, we can offer a lifeline to our digestive system, boosting our overall zest for life. As we sail through the sometimes stormy seas of existence, let's tune into the gentle hum of our inner workings, navigating stress with elegance and perhaps a chuckle or two and maintaining a heartfelt chat with our second brain, delicately steering towards wellness.

5.2 MINDFULNESS AND MEDITATION: TOOLS FOR CALMER DIGESTION

Finding moments of peace can sometimes feel like searching for a needle in a haystack in a world that constantly buzzes with activity. Yet, mindfulness offers a haven, a quiet room within ourselves that we can retreat to, which, in turn, can have profound effects on our digestive health. Mindfulness is the art of being present in the moment, fully engaging with our current experience without judgment or distraction. When applied to stress and digestion, it becomes a powerful tool, transforming our approach to health and well-being.

Mindfulness isn't just about sitting in silence; it's about cultivating an awareness that permeates all aspects of life. This awareness can significantly impact how we manage stress and our gut health. When mindful, we're better equipped to recognize the first signs of stress that might otherwise go unnoticed until they manifest as physical symptoms in our gut.

Meditation Practices

Meditation, a key mindfulness component, offers practical ways to reduce stress and promote digestive health. Here are a few practices that can often be easily integrated into daily life:

- **Focused Breathing**: This involves concentrating on your breath and noticing the air moving in and out of your body, which can help calm the mind and reduce stress.
- **Body Scan Meditation**: Starting from the toes and moving upwards involves paying attention to each part of the body, often revealing areas of tension and allowing them to relax.
- **Mindful Eating**: By eating slowly and savoring each bite,

mindful eating can improve digestion and satiety and even reduce symptoms of gastrointestinal distress.

These practices don't require special equipment or significant amounts of time; they can be incorporated into your routine in just a few minutes daily.

Scientific Evidence

Research has started to shine a light on the tangible benefits of mindfulness and meditation for gut health. Studies have shown that regular meditation can reduce symptoms of IBS, decrease bloating, and improve quality of life. One study published in the *"World Journal of Gastroenterology"* found that participants with IBS who engaged in a mindfulness-based stress reduction program experienced significant relief from their symptoms. This growing body of evidence supports the idea that calming the mind can lead to a calmer digestive system.

Practical Application

Incorporating mindfulness into your daily routine for better gut health can be straightforward. Consider these steps:

- **Start Your Day Mindfully**: Begin with a few minutes of focused breathing each morning to set a calm tone for the day.
- **Pause for Mindful Moments**: Take short breaks to practice mindfulness or focused breathing throughout the day, especially before meals, to encourage mindful eating.
- **Create a Meditation Habit**: Dedicate a specific time each day for meditation, gradually increasing the duration as you become more comfortable with the practice.
- **Use Reminders**: Setting reminders on your phone or

notes around your workspace can help keep mindfulness
at the forefront of your mind.

In weaving mindfulness and meditation into the fabric of our daily lives, we open a pathway to improved digestive health and a more balanced and peaceful existence. These practices invite us to slow down, breathe, and truly inhabit our bodies, counterbalancing modern life's rush and stress. As we nurture this connection with ourselves, we nourish our gut, fostering a sense of well-being that radiates from the inside out.

5.3 MOONLIT MENDING: THE UNSUNG HEROISM OF SNOOZING FOR GUT GLORY

In the hushed whispers of nightfall, a secret healing session is underway, a covert operation led by the sandman himself. When we're lost in our slumber, our bodies, including the bustling metropolis of our gut, get down to the nitty-gritty of repair and restoration. The bond between a blissful night's sleep and a jubilant gut is a tale not told enough, with each chapter influencing the other in a symphony of health and harmony.

The Sleepy Gut Chronicles:

The saga of how sleep and gut health are intertwined is as intricate as it is intriguing. Studies have spotlighted how a twist in our sleep tales can send the gut's microbial community into a tizzy, changing the cast of characters and affecting everything from our immune system's battle strategies to our inflammation narratives.

Conversely, a well-rounded and diverse gut microbiome can be the maestro behind the scenes, orchestrating the production of sleep's leading lights, serotonin, and melatonin, ensuring the show goes smoothly.

But wait, there's more. Skimping on sleep doesn't just leave us cranky; it puts a spanner in the works of digestion, inviting unwelcome guests like constipation or heartburn to the party. It's also prime time for the gut's repair crew to patch any wear and tear, fortifying our defenses against leaky gut syndrome. This underlines the importance of tucking ourselves in for a whole night's encore to support our gut's performance and overall zest for life.

The Art of Sleep Hygiene

Crafting a nocturnal haven and routine that beckons quality shut-eye is key to supporting our gut's health. Consider these sleep hygiene gems:

- **Sticking to a Sleep Schedule**: Like a well-rehearsed dance routine, hitting the hay and rising with the sun regularly keeps our internal rhythm in sync.
- **Setting the Stage:** A cool bedroom, cloaked in darkness and as quiet as a library, creates the perfect backdrop for slumber.
- Evening Encore: Dodge caffeine and rich meals before the curtain call. A light, gut-friendly snack is the ticket if hunger pangs strike.
- **Nightly Rituals**: A pre-bedtime ritual, be it a book chapter, a soak in the tub, or some gentle yoga, whispers to our body that it's time to wind down.

Tales of Tossing and Turning

The plot thickens with the revelation that sleep disorders and gut grievances often share the stage. Ailments like sleep apnea and insomnia can amplify or even spotlight digestive dramas. For instance, the tumultuous breathing of sleep apnea can serenade GERD into action, leaving us with more than just a restless night.

Taking center stage against sleep disorders is crucial for the encore of dreamland and keeping the digestive peace. A duet with health-care maestros can shine a spotlight on solutions, harmonizing sleep and gut health.

Bedtime Stories of Triumph

Let's draw the curtains back on tales of nighttime victories.

Picture a night owl writer, once at odds with IBS, who found inspiration and digestive serenity by embracing the lullabies of a regular sleep schedule. Or envisage a shift worker whose digestive duet was out of tune, finding relief and rhythm by realigning their sleep symphony with the help of a sleep sage.

These narratives are more than mere anecdotes;

They're beacons of hope, showing us the restorative magic woven into the fabric of a good night's sleep. By ensuring we drift off to the land of nod, we're not just resting our weary heads; we're laying the foundation for a gut that's as merry as a lark, ushering in well-being that resonates through every fiber of our being.

5.4 THE SOFTER SIDE OF STAYING SPRY: YOGA AND TAI CHI'S EMBRACE FOR DIGESTIVE DELIGHT

Ah, the modern motto of "go hard or go home," is like telling us to sprint when we really need a leisurely stroll through the park. That's where the gentle embrace of yoga and Tai Chi comes in, like a balm for our often-overlooked digestive system. These aren't your sweat-drenching, muscle-bulging types of exercise. Oh no. They're about nurturing balance and flexibility and ensuring the smooth flow of energy, or Qi, throughout our bodies. This is particularly joyful news for our digestive tracts, which prefer a soft nudge to a hard shove.

The Digestive Ballet

Embracing yoga and Tai Chi is akin to inviting your digestive system to a dance where the movements are gentle, the pace is steady, and the focus is on enjoying the rhythm. These practices offer a tender massage to our insides, boosting blood flow to the digestive organs and encouraging our meals to mosey on through without a hitch. They're the antidote to the bloating, gas, and constipation that often plague us when stress and sedentary lifestyles take their toll. Plus, the profound, mindful breathing cornerstone is like a lullaby to stress, lulling it to sleep and letting our guts get on with their business in peace.

Yoga's Digestive Serenades

Certain yoga poses are like love songs for our digestive system, each designed to stimulate, stretch, and soothe. Here are a few hits from the digestive chart-toppers:

- **Apanasana (Wind-Relieving Pose):** A cozy hug of the knees to the chest that says, "There, there" to trapped gas and bloating.
- **Pavanamuktasana (Knees-to-Chest Pose):** A gentle squeeze that whispers sweet nothings to our bowels, encouraging them to let go of what doesn't serve us.
- **Twists:** A soft wringing out of the torso that's less about wringing out the laundry and more about inviting toxins to kindly exit stage left.
- **Forward Bends:** A polite nudge to the abdomen, encouraging digestion to keep moving along.

As with any good relationship, listening and responding with kindness is essential. If a pose feels more like a drama than a romance, it's okay to skip it and find one that feels like a better match.

Tai Chi's Gentle Flow

With its graceful, flowing movements, Tai Chi is less about breaking a sweat and more about fostering inner calm – a sort of meditation in motion. It's the slow dance of the exercise world, where each movement is deliberate and mindful. This dance reduces stress and lights a spark for better digestion. The deep, abdominal breathing is a love letter to the 'rest and digest' system, setting the stage for a tranquil digestive process.

Embarking on Your Journey

Stepping into the world of yoga and Tai Chi might feel like learning a new language, but here are some friendly nudges to get you started:

- Seek out beginner or gentle classes focusing on nurturing rather than conquering.
- The internet is a treasure trove of resources – from YouTube tutorials to online classes, there's a guide for every level of curiosity.
- Remember, this is a dialogue with your body. If something feels off, there's no shame in modifying or simply taking a rest.
- Consistency is your companion on this journey. A little bit every day can do wonders compared to a once-a-week marathon session.

Inviting yoga and Tai Chi into our daily routine is a gentle yet powerful way to honor our digestive system. It's a reminder that sometimes, the most profound healing comes not from pushing ourselves to the limit but from moving with intention and grace. So, let's roll out our mats or step into our Tai Chi stance and give our guts the loving attention they deserve, one breath and one movement at a time.

5.5 SOCIAL CONNECTIONS: HOW RELATIONSHIPS INFLUENCE OUR GUT

Our ties with family, friends, and the broader community do more than just enrich our lives with joy and companionship. They also weave a protective web around our gut health, buffering against the erosive effects of stress. This section explores the intricate ways in which our social bonds can be a balm for our digestive well-being.

Social Health and the Gut

Picture your gut as a serene ecosystem thriving under the right conditions. Stress, however, can be likened to a storm that disrupts this tranquility. Social interactions act as a calming force, mitigating stress and fostering an environment where our digestive system can flourish. Engaging with others triggers the release of oxytocin, often dubbed the 'love hormone,' which not only makes us feel good but also dampens stress and its adverse effects on the gut. This hormonal surge can soothe inflammation and improve gut motility, illustrating the profound impact of our social connections on our digestive health.

Support Systems

Having a network of supportive relationships is akin to possessing a well-stocked toolkit for managing life's ups and downs. When stress threatens to overwhelm us, these bonds offer emotional scaffolding, helping us navigate rough times. This support is invaluable for maintaining gut health, providing a buffer against stress-induced digestive issues. Whether it's a heartfelt conversation with a friend or a comforting hug from a loved one, these interactions can significantly lower our stress levels, offering a protective shield for our gut.

Community Engagement

For those seeking to bolster their gut health through social means, engaging with a community centered on wellness can be particularly rewarding. Here are ways to connect:

- **Joining Health-focused Groups:** Whether it's a yoga class, a meditation group, or a cooking club focused on nutritious eating, participating in these communities can foster not only new skills but also meaningful connections.
- **Volunteering:** Giving back to the community can provide a sense of purpose and reduce feelings of isolation, both of which are beneficial for stress management and, by extension, gut health.
- **Online Support Networks:** For those with specific health conditions, online forums and support groups offer a space to share experiences, tips, and encouragement, creating a virtual community of care.

Real-life Impacts

Consider the story of Anna, who, after being diagnosed with a chronic digestive disorder, felt isolated and stressed, exacerbating her symptoms. Upon joining a local support group for individuals with similar conditions, she found valuable advice and a sense of belonging. This newfound community played a crucial role in her stress management strategy, leading to noticeable improvements in her symptoms.

Then there's Miguel, a retiree who took up volunteering at a community garden. The social interactions and physical activity involved in tending to the garden significantly reduced his stress levels, positively affecting his digestive health. These stories underscore the decisive role that social connections and community engagement can play in fostering gut health.

In wrapping up, it's clear that our gut health is inextricably linked to the quality of our social connections. The evidence is compelling, from the calming effects of oxytocin released during interactions to the stress-buffering support of our social networks. Engaging with our community and nurturing meaningful relationships can be a tonic for our digestive system, highlighting the importance of social bonds in our overall wellness strategy.

As we move forward, let's carry with us the understanding that our social world is not just a backdrop to our lives but a vital component of our health, influencing our well-being in profound and lasting ways. This realization opens up new avenues for enhancing our health, emphasizing the power of connection, community, and care in our journey toward wellness.

SUMMARY AND HOMEWORK ACTION PLAN

Imagine you're in your favorite cozy corner, the world's hustle and bustle a mere whisper behind closed doors. But then, whoosh! Stress barges in, scattering peace like autumn leaves in a gust. This uninvited chaos, my friends, mirrors what happens in the secret garden of our gut when stressed and decides to throw a party. It's not just our sleep that's interrupted; our digestive system gets jittery, trying to keep up with stress's vigorous dance steps.

Action Steps:

- **Move Joyfully:** Embrace activities that spark joy, whether a brisk walk or shaking your groove in the living room.
- **Breathe Deeply:** Try diaphragmatic breathing to calm the internal storms, offering peace to your gut.
- **Embrace Nature:** Spend time in green spaces; even a little pottering in the garden can soothe the soul and the stomach.
- **Watch Your Bites and Sips:** Consider easing on caffeine and sugary delights that can turn the stress dial a notch.
- **Begin the Day with Intent:** Start with mindful breathing to set a calm tone.
- **Savor Your Meals:** Eat slowly, enjoying each bite, to honor your body and its digestive journey.
- **Meditate Daily:** Carve out a moment for meditation, building a sanctuary of calm in your day.
- **Craft a Sleep Ritual:** Establish a soothing pre-sleep routine to signal your body to wind down.
- **Create a Sleep Haven:** Make your bedroom a sanctuary of sleep, cool, dark, and quiet.
- **Mind Your Diet:** Opt for light, gut-friendly evening snacks if needed, steering clear of late-night feasting.
- **Find Your Flow:** Explore the movement of beginning yoga or Tai C classes.
- **Listen to Your Body:** Embrace good poses and movements, adjusting as needed.
- **Consistency is Key:** Daily practice nurtures your gut and soothes your spirit.
- **Reach Out:** Engage with friends, family, and communities that lift you.
- **Volunteer:** Lend a hand where needed, finding purpose and connection.

- **Join Supportive Circles:** Find groups that share your wellness journey online or in person.

In wrapping up this chapter, let's carry the wisdom that managing stress, embracing mindfulness, cherishing sleep, moving gently, and fostering connections aren't just acts of self-care; they're serenades to our gut. As we navigate life's ebbs and flows, let's do so with grace, humor, and an unwavering commitment to our digestive health, dancing through life's storms with our heads held high and our bellies at ease.

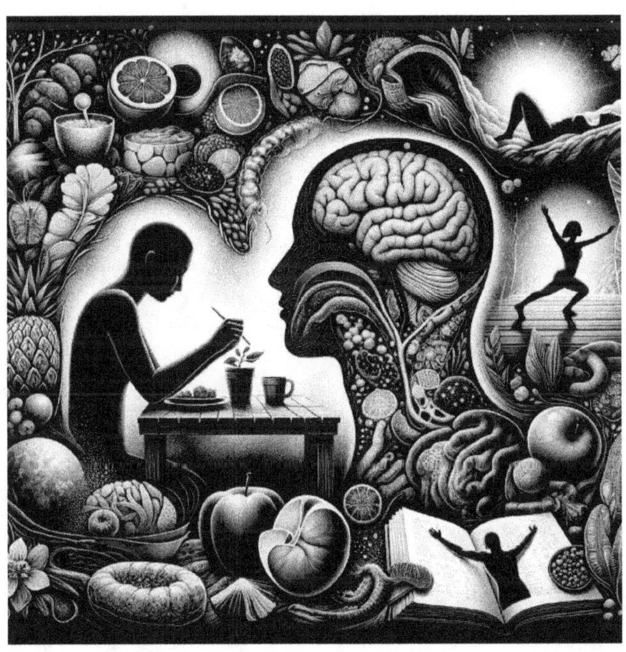

IN RHYTHM WITH YOUR GUT: MOVING TOWARDS DIGESTIVE HEALTH

Imagine this: It's early morning, the dew's still fresh on the grass, whispering, "Wake up, love." It's as if the earth is stretching gently, urging you to do the same. Now, I'm not one to leap out of bed at the crack of dawn anymore, but there's wisdom in syncing up with the world's natural rhythms. Just like a good morning stretch can shake off sleep, some exercise can do wonders for a sleepy digestive system, infusing it with energy and balance.

EXERCISE AND MICROBIOME

Now, scientists (bless their curious hearts) have uncovered something remarkable. Our gut, that bustling city of microbes we carry around, thrives on a bit of physical hustle. It turns out that lacing up those walking shoes or unrolling the yoga mat does more than keep your heart young; it cultivates a lush microbial garden in your gut.

Diversity is the spice of life, leading to smoother digestion, less inflammation, and a lower chance of those pesky chronic illnesses.

How Exercise Tickles Your Gut Flora

Engaging in physical activity increases butyrate — think of it as a superfood for your gut cells, keeping the walls of your intestines strong and inflammation at bay.

The Evidence

A peek into the journal "Gut" reveals that folks who regularly break a sweat have a more diverse community of gut residents than those who prefer a more sedentary lifestyle. Quite the incentive to get moving.

Types of Beneficial Exercise

Now, not all exercises are born equal in the eyes of your gut. Some are like fine dining for your microbes:

Aerobic Activities: Whether it's a brisk walk, a leisurely bike ride, or a swim, these activities get the blood pumping and the digestive tract moving more efficiently.

Yoga: It's not just about bending and breathing; those twists are like internal massages for your organs, keeping things moving smoothly.

Pilates: A strong core isn't just for looks; it supports your digestive system too, from your pelvic floor to those deep belly muscles.

Exercise Recommendations

The secret sauce to benefiting your gut is finding that sweet spot of exercise frequency and intensity:

Ease Into It: Starting slow is my motto. There's no rush in the journey to wellness.

A Dab'll Do Ya: Regular, moderate exercise beats sporadic, intense sessions. It's the long game that counts.

Heed Your Body's Whispers: Not every exercise suits everybody. Listen closely and adjust as needed.

SCIENTIFIC NODS

This isn't just old wives' tales; the science backs it up. Studies from fancy titles like the "International Journal of Sports Nutrition and Exercise Metabolism" confirm that moderate exercise enriches our gut flora diversity, akin to winning the health lottery.

Moreover, the "American Journal of Gastroenterology" notes that those regular moves can soothe IBS symptoms, a nod to exercise's power in the digestive dance.

Incorporating exercise into our daily routine is akin to greeting the dawn with open arms. It's about creating harmony within, letting every stretch and step bring our digestive health into a delightful equilibrium with the rest of our being.

By embracing the dynamic duo of movement and microbiome, we step closer to a life filled with vitality, where every day is an opportunity to dance in rhythm with our gut.

Mindful Walking

Now, let's add a sprinkle of mindfulness to our walking pie. Turning your walk into a "now" experience reduces stress, which, in turn, keeps your gut from throwing tantrums. Here's how to walk mindfully:

Feel Your Feet: Notice the kiss of each footfall on the earth.

Breathe in Sync: Let your breath find its rhythm with your strides.

Embrace Your Surroundings: Let the world's colors and sounds envelop you, gently nudging your thoughts back when they wander.

6.3 STRENGTH TRAINING: BUILDING A STRONGER DIGESTIVE SYSTEM

When we chat about boosting our gut health, pumping iron might not be the first thing that pops into your head. Yet, here I am, ready to tell you that hoisting a few weights around could do as much for your insides as it does for your biceps. Strength training isn't just about sculpting those muscles or shedding the extra pudding; it's also about jazzing up your digestive system.

Strength Training and the Gut

Diving into some strength training does wonders, not just for your physique but for your belly's well-being too. Let's peek at the perks:

Sprightlier Bowel Movements: Some strength work tightens up those abdominal and pelvic floor muscles, essential for smooth sailing in the bathroom department. This becomes a gold mine as we age and those muscles start to think about retiring.

Metabolism on Fire: Muscle mass from lifting weights puts your metabolism on speedy mode, meaning you're burning calories even while you're knitting or reading. A bustling metabolism helps keep the weight in check, warding off those gut troubles tied to obesity.

A Dose of Happy: Strength training sends those endorphins soaring, cutting down stress, which, if you didn't know, can throw a wrench in your gut health. Less stress equals a happier tummy.

Safety First

If you're eyeing the weights and thinking, "Where do I start?" or you're in the golden years category like me, here's how to keep it safe:

Seek Expertise: New to the weight room? Chatting with a personal trainer can set you on the right path, showing you the ropes without mishaps.

Form Over Fuss: Keep an eye on making each move right, even with lighter weights. It's about engaging the right muscles without causing trouble.

Listen to Your Body's Whispers: A bit of muscle tenderness is part of the game, but any sharp pains are your body's way of saying, "Hold on a minute!"

Home Gym Hacks

No gym membership? No worries. You can still get your strength training in with things you've got lying around the house:

Bodyweight Bonanza: Squats, push-ups, and planks don't need anything but you. Plus, they're splendid for starting strength training.

Resistance Bands: Stretchy and easy to stash away, these bands can spice up your workout with various exercises.

DIY Weights: Water bottles or cans of beans can double as dumbbells for those bicep curls or shoulder presses.

Chair Chores: Chairs aren't just for sitting; use them for dips or seated leg lifts, perfect for adding strength work without needing to stand.

Keeping Tabs

Watching your progress isn't just motivating; it's enlightening, especially when you're tracking the changes in your gut health too:

Workout Diary: Jot down what you do, the weights you lift, and how many times. Pair this with any notes on your gut's feeling to see the connection.

Symptom Spotting: Keep an eye on how your digestive system responds in a diary. You might start seeing patterns that show you're on the right track.

Snapshots and Sizing: Outer changes might be subtle, but keeping visual and measurement records can be a great motivator and a way to see the impact on your overall health.

Incorporating strength training into your routine isn't just a boon for your muscles; it's also a cheerleader for your gut health. It's a holistic approach to keeping fit, proving that a bit of weightlifting can support your strength and your digestive harmony. With a pinch of safety, a dash of creativity in your work-outs, and a commitment to keeping an eye on your progress, strength training can be a formidable ally in your journey to a vibrant gut. So, why not give it a lift?

6.4 THE ROLE OF HYDRATION IN EXERCISE AND DIGESTION

In the grand tapestry of maintaining a vibrant digestive system, hydration emerges as a vital thread, interwoven intricately with the fabric of our overall health. Much like a river nourishes the land through which it flows, adequate water intake sustains our bodies, catalyzing crucial processes that keep us functioning at our peak. This is particularly true regarding exercise and digestion, where water plays dual pivotal roles as both facilitators and guardians of our well-being.

Hydration Essentials

Water's influence stretches far and wide, touching every aspect of our physiological landscape. In the realm of exercise, it acts as the ultimate performance enhancer, regulating body temperature, lubricating joints, and transporting nutrients to provide energy and keep our systems in harmony. As for digestion, water is the cornerstone of the entire process. It aids in breaking down food, allowing nutrients to be absorbed more efficiently, and prevents constipation by softening stools, ensuring a smooth journey through the intestines.

Hydration Essentials

Imagine your body as a sophisticated tea party, where every guest —your organs—needs the perfect amount of tea to keep the conversation lively. Too little, and the party dulls; too much, and it's chaos. Water is the maestro in physical exertion and the grand digestive ballet, conducting an orchestra of bodily functions with grace and precision. It keeps your joints jumping and your digestive tract trotting along happily.

Fluid Intake Guidelines

Now, the golden question: How much of this liquid gold should one drink? While the adage suggests a daily eight-glass waltz, the dance varies with the dancer. Your rhythm—a brisk walk in the park or a tango in the summer heat—and the weather's tune and your body's unique melody dictate your hydration needs.

Before Exercise: Drink about 17-20 ounces of water two to three hours before you start your workout. This gives your body ample time to process the fluid and prepare for sweat loss.

During Exercise: Aim to sip 7-10 ounces every 10-20 minutes during your activity. The goal is to replace fluids as you lose them through sweat.

After Exercise: Replenish with approximately 16-24 ounces of water for every pound lost during the workout. Weighing yourself before and after can help gauge this loss more accurately.

Signs of Dehydration

Staying vigilant for dehydration's telltale signs ensures we can swiftly rebalance our fluid levels. These indicators serve as our body's distress signals, prompting us to replenish and restore:

Thirst: Though seemingly obvious, you're already mildly dehydrated when you're thirsty.

Urine Color: Light, straw-colored urine indicates good hydration, while dark yellow or amber suggests dehydration.

Fatigue and Dizziness: A lack of fluids can lead to feelings of tiredness and sometimes even lightheadedness.

Dry Mouth and Lips: This is one of the earliest signs your body needs more water.

Addressing these symptoms promptly by increasing your water intake can help prevent further dehydration, which, if left unchecked, can severely impact both exercise performance and digestive health.

Electrolytes and Hydration

Electrolytes, the minerals in our blood and other body fluids that carry an electric charge, are crucial players in the hydration game. They include sodium, potassium, calcium, and magnesium and are essential for balancing the amount of water in your body, moving nutrients into your cells, and moving wastes out of them. During exercise, especially in hot weather or during long sessions, we lose these vital minerals through sweat. Replenishing them is critical to maintaining fluid balance and preventing dehydration.

Here's how to ensure you're getting enough:

Dietary Sources: Incorporating foods rich in electrolytes into your diet is a natural way to replenish these minerals. Bananas and oranges are excellent for potassium, dairy products for calcium, nuts, and seeds for magnesium, and table salt for sodium.

Electrolyte Solutions: For intense exercise exceeding an hour or for those who sweat heavily, electrolyte-enhanced waters or sports drinks can be helpful. These solutions are formulated to replace lost minerals efficiently.

Supplementation: In some cases, electrolyte supplements may be necessary for individuals with specific health conditions or dietary restrictions.

Consulting with a healthcare provider can help determine if this route is appropriate.

Keeping the river of life flowing with the right mix of water and electrolytes ensures you're hitting the right notes in exercise and digestion and keeps the party going inside you, vibrant and joyous. So, let's raise a glass (of water) to a life well-hydrated and full of zest!

6.5. OVERCOMING BARRIERS: TIPS FOR STAYING ACTIVE IN LATER LIFE

The twilight years, when the spirit is willing, the flesh has developed a rather inconvenient sense of humor. Engaging in bodily frolic can feel like negotiating with a temperamental antique clock —utterly delightful when it chimes but occasionally stubborn and resistant to winding. Yet, let me assure you, embarking on the quest for an active lifestyle amidst the golden haze of later life is not only possible; it's a recipe for a joyously ticking body and a flourishing gut garden.

Challenges to Staying Active: A Humorous Glance

Let's face it, the body in its senior edition comes with its own set of quirks:

- **Physical Limitations:** Suddenly, the marathon runner within us is considering a new career in competitive sitting. Mobility might ebb, and chronic conditions could send us memos to slow down.
- **Fear of Injury**: The ground has gotten further away, hasn't it? The fear of taking a tumble or stirring up the dust in old health issues can make one eye the yoga mat suspiciously.
- **Lack of Energy:** Some days, exercise is as appealing as climbing Everest in slippers. Less activity breeds less energy—a vicious cycle that's as hard to kick as a midnight biscuit habit.
- **Isolation:** Without a partner in crime, embarking on physical feats can seem as daunting as solo karaoke.

Adaptable Exercise Options: There's More Than One Way to Knead Dough

Fear not, for every creaky joint, there's a workaround:

- **Chair Yoga:** Who says you can't do yoga and be seated simultaneously? Perfect for those of us whose balance is more "vintage" than "vinyasa."
- **Water Aerobics**: It's like being a graceful swan in a pond if swans are particularly keen on joint health and resistance training.

- **Low-Impact Walking:** Stroll like you're perusing the aisles of nostalgia, perhaps with a fancy stick or a sturdy arm to lean on.
- **Resistance Band Exercises:** These bands are the unsung heroes of the exercise world—portable, versatile, and less likely to cause mischief than dumbbells.

Motivation Strategies: Lighting the Sparkler Underneath

- **Set Realistic Goals:** Consider it plotting a gentle rebellion against inertia. Small victories pave the way to grand adventures.
- **Find Activities You Enjoy:** If dancing in the living room or tending to a riotous garden brings joy, who's to say it's not the best kind of exercise?
- **Buddy Up:** A partner in mild exertion can turn exercise into a social hour, minus the tea and scones.
- **Celebrate Progress:** Every step, every stretch, deserves applause—perhaps even a tiny, self-congratulatory pastry (for energy, of course).

Community Resources: The Quest for Companionship and Adventure

The world is teeming with opportunities for the energetically seasoned:

- **Senior Centers and Clubs:** Where camaraderie meets calisthenics, and exercise often comes with a side of gossip.
- **Local Parks and Recreation:** The great outdoors is an open invitation for walks, talks, and perhaps a discreet game of tag.

- **Online Platforms:** Bringing the world to your living room, one click at a time. Who knew one could travel the globe and get fit without leaving the couch?
- **Volunteer Opportunities:** Lend a hand, move your feet, and fill your heart—physical activity with purpose is doubly rewarding.

As we curtain this chapter, let's remember: staying active in our silver and gold years isn't about outrunning Father Time; it's about inviting him for a gentle jog or a merry waltz. It's about nurturing our inner ecosystems with every chuckle-inducing stretch and every life-affirming step. Onward to the next chapter, where the mysteries of the gut await us, ripe for exploration like a farmers' market of scientific wonders. Let's savor each discovery, each nugget of knowledge, like a fine wine or a perfectly aged cheese, enriching our journey towards health, happiness, and perhaps a bit of cheeky defiance against the aging process.

SUMMARY AND ACTION PLAN: IN RHYTHM WITH YOUR GUT: MOVING TOWARDS DIGESTIVE HEALTH

Chapter 6 focuses on the integral role of exercise in maintaining and improving digestive health through its positive impact on the gut microbiome. It highlights various exercises beneficial for digestive health, including aerobic activities, yoga, and Pilates, each contributing uniquely to the body's overall well-being. The chapter emphasizes starting exercise routines slowly, listening to the body's needs, and gradually increasing intensity and frequency for optimal gut health benefits.

- **Exercise and the Microbiome**: Exercise stimulates the gut flora, enhancing digestive efficiency and overall health.

- **Beneficial Exercises:** Aerobic activities improve blood circulation and gut movement, yoga is an internal massage, and Pilates strengthens core muscles supporting the digestive system.
- **Exercise Recommendations**: Start slowly, adjust to your body's needs, and incorporate exercise into daily life for harmony.
- **Strength Training:** Benefits include improved bowel movements, a boosted metabolism, and reduced stress, contributing to better gut health.
- **Hydration:** Essential for exercise and digestion, with guidelines provided for before, during, and after exercise to prevent dehydration.
- **Overcoming Barriers:** Offers solutions for staying active in later life, addressing physical limitations, fear of injury, lack of energy, and isolation, with a focus on adaptable exercise options and motivation strategies.

Action Plan for Readers

Identify Your Starting Point:

- Assess your current physical activity and digestive health level to personalize your approach.

Incorporate Beneficial Exercises:

- Begin with low-impact aerobic activities like walking or swimming.
- Add gentle yoga or Pilates sessions to your routine, focusing on movements that support digestive health.
- Gradually introduce strength training exercises, starting with bodyweight exercises or resistance bands.

Hydration:

- Follow the hydration guidelines before, during, and after exercise to maintain optimal digestive health.
- Incorporate foods rich in electrolytes to support hydration.

Overcome Barriers:

- Address physical limitations by choosing low-impact or chair-based exercises.
- Mitigate fear of injury by seeking guidance from fitness professionals and focusing on form.
- Boost energy levels with short, enjoyable activities and gradually increasing intensity.
- Combat isolation by joining group classes or online communities focused on fitness and wellness.

Track Your Progress:

- Keep a diary of your exercise routines, noting how your body and digestive system respond.
- Monitor symptoms and improvements in digestive health to adjust your routine as needed.

Stay Motivated:

- Set realistic, achievable goals for both exercise and digestive health improvements.
- Celebrate progress, no matter how small, and consider partnering with a friend or joining a community for support.

Consult Healthcare Providers:

- Before starting any new exercise regimen, especially if you have existing health conditions, consult a healthcare provider for personalized advice.

Following this action plan, readers can embark on a journey toward improved digestive health through exercise, hydration, and mindful practices, adjusting their approach based on personal needs and progress.

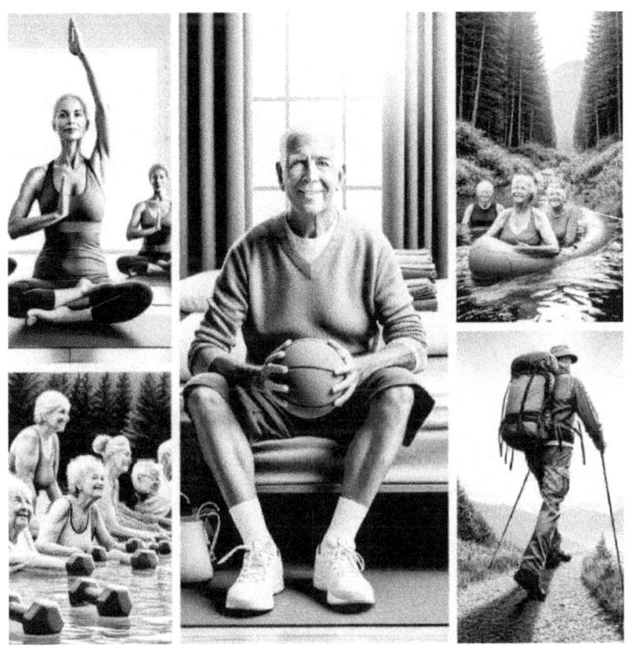

THE NEW FRONTIER OF GUT HEALTH

Picture this: you're meandering through a bustling farmers' market with the promise of discovering hidden treasures around every corner. You snag a bite of crisp apple here, a dollop of golden honey there - each taste a tiny expedition. This, my dear, is the thrill of the chase in microbiome research. Scientists, those intrepid explorers, are delving into the wilderness of our innards, unearthing secrets buried in our belly's depths. Each revelation is a potential game-changer in the grand scheme of our well-being. It's an exhilarating era, with every research paper serving up delectable insights into the intricate ecosystem that resides within us.

7.1 THE FRONTIER OF MICROBIOME RESEARCH: WHAT'S NEXT?

Innovative Research Methods

Imagine if, in your quest for understanding the secrets of a masterpiece painting, you swapped your old, trusty magnifying glass for a state-of-the-art, high-def, 3D-imaging spectroscope. That's the kind of technological wizardry microbiome researchers are wielding nowadays. We're talking next-generation sequencing and computational models so advanced they could give Nostradamus a run for his money, predicting the future of our gut health with startling accuracy. It's like having a crystal ball but for your belly.

Potential Discoveries

Envision a future where mapping someone's gut microbiome is as routine as taking their temperature. We're on the brink of such discoveries, possibly uncovering bacterial species flying under our radar yet playing pivotal roles in our health. Fancy finding a little bugger that can tweak your mood faster than a shot of espresso, or one that fine-tunes nutrient absorption, ensuring every morsel you eat is transformed into precisely what your body craves. It's like having a personal nutritionist hidden in your microbiome.

Microbiome and Diseases

The saga of our gut bacteria and their link to diseases unfolds like a mystery novel with plot twists. Research is revealing connections between our gut buddies and a host of ailments - from Alzheimer's to diabetes, heart disease to cancer. It's as though we've uncovered a secret network of passages connecting distant, seemingly unrelated realms. Grasping these links hands us the key to groundbreaking treatments and prevention strategies that start with our gut. Imagine tweaking your microbiome to fend off mental health issues - a whole new world of therapeutic possibilities served up on a silver platter.

Future Therapies

The next big thing in medicine is lurking in our guts, of all places. Fecal microbiota transplantation (FMT) is already a thing, believe it or not, using healthy donor poop to give someone's gut flora a makeover. And that's just for starters. The research labs are abuzz with the potential of precision probiotics - bespoke bacterial blends crafted to fix you up, targeting specific health concerns. Pop a capsule, and poof! Your personalized gut flora gets to work, fine-tuning your health, mood, and even your dietary quirks.

Embarking on this voyage into the new frontiers of gut health isn't merely a scientific expedition; it's a deeply personal odyssey. As we peel back the layers of the microbiome's influence on our well-being, we're handed the reins to steer our health destiny through diet, lifestyle, and, perhaps, the magic of future therapies. The breakthroughs waiting in the wings promise to flip the script on our health narrative and hand us the tools for a tailor-made approach to wellness, nurturing our inner ecosystem to flourish like never before.

7.2 PERSONALIZED NUTRITION: TAILORING DIET TO YOUR GUT'S NEEDS

Well, let's chat about this fancy notion of personalized nutrition, shall we? Picture this: a chef and a nutritionist conspiring in the kitchen, crafting a menu that's not just about whether you're a fan of Brussels sprouts or would rather eat cardboard than tofu. No, they're delving deep into the nitty-gritty of your gut's unique flora and fauna. It's as if your digestive tract had its own dietary consultant, ensuring every morsel you munch on is a match made in heaven for your microbiota. We're stepping out of the era of one-size-fits-all eating guides and into a world where your dinner plate is as bespoke as a tailor-made suit.

Technological Advances

Now, wait to get me started on the wizardry that's making all this possible. We've got artificial intelligence and machine learning playing detective with the data from our gut bugs, diets, and how well we fare health-wise. We have a crystal ball that can predict how your tummy will react to a slice of apple pie or a kale smoothie, tweaking your eating plan on the fly. And here you thought "The Jetsons" was futuristic!

Benefits for Individuals

The perks of this culinary customization are nothing to sneeze at. Imagine fine-tuning your food intake to get the nutrients your body craves, turning you into a well-oiled machine. Say goodbye to those after-lunch energy slumps and hello to a version of you that's energized, healthier, possibly even a bit slimmer. It's like having a secret map to the treasure trove of optimal health designed just for you.

Challenges and Considerations

But, as with all great adventures, there are dragons to slay along the way. First, we must keep a tight lid on our personal health info. In the wrong hands, it could lead to a pickle or two.

Then there's the matter of the price tag of getting your gut's dossier – not everyone can afford such luxuries, potentially leaving some folks in the dust. And let's not forget, we're still pretty much in kindergarten when it comes to understanding our microbiome. Plus, there's a whole can of ethical worms – could this data affect your health insurance or job prospects?

Despite these hurdles, the journey toward personalized nutrition is like peering through a kaleidoscope into the future of food and health. It's a future where eating plans are as individual as fingerprints, ushering in a new dawn of disease prevention and peak health tailored just for you. As we unravel the mysteries of our microbiome and technology races ahead, the dream of a diet designed just for you is becoming increasingly a reality. Here's to a future where we all get to eat our cake and have it too, perfectly portioned to our personal gut health, of course!

7.3 THE PROMISE OF PROBIOTICS: NEXT-GENERATION SUPPLEMENTS

Let's gossip about probiotics, those tiny but mighty allies in our quest for gut harmony. Picture them as the dependable pals of our internal ecosystem, akin to a garden where they're the bees buzzing about, ensuring everything's in apple-pie order. But, as we've learned, not all these microscopic chums are cut from the same cloth. Oh no, we've journeyed from the simplistic days of yogurt starters to the brave new world of tailored, strain-specific supplements, each with its secret handshake with our health.

Evolution of Probiotics

Our tale of probiotics starts with a nod to the past, where fermented foods were not just culinary delights but bearers of gut wisdom, passed down through generations like a cherished family recipe. Then came the leap – from kraut and kefir to the first wave of probiotic supplements, a giant step towards bottling those benefits. Initially, these were like the variety packs of bacteria, a bit of this, a bit of that, with a hopeful glance towards better gut health.

But as the plot thickened, with science delving deeper into the gut's mysteries, we discovered that the magic of probiotics lies in their diversity. Each strain, it turns out, is a specialist focused on particular health gigs – from soothing the irritable bowels to lifting our spirits. This revelation ushered in the era of next-generation probiotics and bespoke concoctions aimed at specific ailments, showcasing the finesse of our growing understanding.

Strain-Specific Benefits

The crux of the matter with probiotics is this notion of strain specificity. It's like having an orchestra in your gut – each microbe plays a different instrument, contributing to the symphony of your health. For instance, Lactobacillus rhamnosus GG, a virtuoso in its own right, tackles diarrhea with aplomb, while Bifidobacterium longum 35624 takes a bow for its role in quelling irritable bowel syndrome. It's clear, then, that picking the right probiotic isn't a game of eeny, meeny, miny, moe but a thoughtful selection of your health allies.

Innovations in Delivery Systems

The journey of these tiny warriors from the bottle to the bowel is fraught with peril, thanks to the acidic gauntlet of the stomach. Herein lies the rub: how do we escort them safely to their destination? Science, ever the ingenious, has concocted solutions such as microencapsulation, a fancy term for giving our bacterial buddies a suit of armor against stomach acid. Then there's the dynamic duo of probiotics and prebiotics, or synbiotics, ensuring safe passage and a warm welcome in the gut, fostering a thriving microbial metropolis.

Regulatory and Quality Concerns

With the probiotic market blooming, the thorny issue of quality and regulation comes to the fore. The landscape here is as varied as a patchwork quilt, with some regions treating probiotics as mere dietary supplements while others bestow upon them the gravitas of medicinal products. This discrepancy begs the question: How do we ensure what's on the label is what's in the jar and that these microscopic hitchhikers remain hale and hearty until their expiration date?

Advances in genetic sequencing and microbiological testing are the lighthouses guiding us through these murky waters, offering more precise methods to verify the identity and vitality of these probiotic populations. Furthermore, the call for standardized production and storage protocols is loud and clear, ensuring these beneficial bacteria aren't undone by heat, humidity, or time trials.

As we march forward, the evolution of probiotic supplements from humble beginnings to their current state-of-the-art incarnations is a testament to our journey of discovery in gut health. With each scientific breakthrough and regulatory stride, we inch closer to fulfilling the full potential of probiotics as cornerstones of our well-being, ensuring this chapter in health and nutrition is not just a passing trend but a lasting legacy.

7.4 GUT HEALTH AND LONGEVITY: EXTENDING QUALITY OF LIFE

Now, let's cha-cha into the fascinating world of gut health and its tango with aging. You see, having a gut bustling with the right kind of bacteria isn't just about dodging those awkward digestive moments; it's about laying down the red carpet for a future that's not just longer but sparkles with zest and vigor. The secret potion for a life that stretches gracefully into the golden years might be swirling around in our bellies.

The Relationship Between Gut Health and Aging

In the latest gossip from the science world, our guts are getting all the limelight, and rightly so. The mix and harmony of our gut buddies can make or break how gracefully we age. A harmonious gut sings a tune of reduced inflammation, keeping those age-related gremlins at bay. But let the balance tip, and you're looking at a body that's a bit too eager to show its age, rolling out the welcome mat for unwelcome guests like Alzheimer's, heart disease, and osteoporosis. So, it's not just about avoiding a tummy ache; it's about curating a body built to last.

Dietary and Lifestyle Interventions for Longevity

Embarking on the quest for a life well-lived? The magic starts on your plate. A smorgasbord of fiber-rich foods feeds the excellent gut critters, while fermented goodies like yogurt and sauerkraut give them a leg up. And let's not forget the power of shaking a leg or striking a yoga pose to sprinkle some diversity into our microbial mix. A dash of meditation and a good night's sleep also do wonders for the gut, laying the bricks for a long and fulfilling path.

Unveiling Recent Research Findings

The buzz about gut health and longevity isn't just talk. A treasure trove of research is now backing up the claim that a diverse gut gang means a ticket to a longer, sprightlier life. Revelations include bacteria that could shield our brains from the sands of time, hinting at ways to keep our minds sharp as tacks as the years tick by. These knowledge nuggets underscore the gut's starring role in the saga of our lifespan and the quality of our twilight years.

Peering Into the Future of Anti-Aging Research

Peeking over the horizon, the future of dodging the wrinkles and creaks looks promising, with our gut flora in the leading role. Scientists are busy bees exploring how tweaking our gut guests with diet, probiotics, and even more avant-garde methods could add candles to the birthday cake and keep our wits about us and our joints jiving. The dream of concocting microbiome-based elixirs to fend off the ticking clock is inching closer to reality, heralding a new chapter where living longer also means living fuller.

As we dive deeper into the mysteries of the gut microbiome, it's becoming crystal clear that the fountain of youth is nestled within our insides. With every breakthrough, we're reminded that pampering our gut is more than a mere act of self-care; it's a long-term investment in a future where we can dance into the sunset with vitality and verve as our dance partners. Here's to a journey that's not just about adding years to our lives but life to our years, all thanks to the little world thriving inside us.

7.5 BEYOND DIGESTION: THE GUT'S ROLE IN IMMUNE FUNCTION

Now, let's waltz beyond the realm of digestion and peek into the gut's role in our immune system, which is far more than just a bystander in our body's health saga. Picture your gut as the unsung hero, quietly orchestrating the ebb and flow of your immune response, a bit like a conductor with a bacterial orchestra at their fingertips.

Gut-Immune System Interaction

Imagine your gut as a teeming metropolis, bustling with microbial inhabitants that chat up the immune system's cells. These aren't just casual coffee shop talks; they're vital discussions that help prep your immune system to discern friend from foe. Beneficial gut bacteria are the diplomats, issuing compounds that quell inflammation and pep-talk the immune cells into top form. It's a well-oiled machine designed to keep things running smoothly without causing a ruckus.

Microbiome Imbalances and Immunity

But, when the microbial balance tips, it's like throwing a wrench in the works. Dysbiosis, or this imbalance, can lead to a bit of a tizzy within your immune system, making you more prone to infections and prompting it to start a bit of friendly fire on its tissues. It's akin to the chaos a city's gridlock, where messages get jumbled, leading to overreactions or no reaction.

Probiotics and Immune Health

But fear not, for probiotics are the cavalry coming to the rescue. These friendly microbes act as the peacekeepers, mending broken lines of communication within the gut's ecosystem. Specific strains from the Lactobacillus and Bifidobacterium families are like the special agents boosting your body's defense forces, helping to fend off those pesky invaders more efficiently. They're the unsung heroes bolstering our defenses against the sniffles and tummy troubles.

Holistic Health Strategies

To keep this dynamic duo of gut and immune health in tip-top shape, consider a holistic game plan:

- **Diverse Diet**: Feast on a kaleidoscope of fiber-packed foods to keep your microbial city vibrant and diverse.
- **Regular Probiotic Intake:** Regularly invite probiotic-rich foods to the party or pop a probiotic supplement to keep the peace within.
- **Stress Management:** Keep stress in check, lest it throws a spanner in your gut's works. Yoga, knitting, or whatever floats your boat can help keep the peace.
- **Adequate Sleep:** Catch those Z's to keep your gut inhabitants happy and your immune system ready for battle.

As we delve deeper into the mysteries of our gut, it's clear it plays a starring role in our body's defense strategy. By looking after our gut through mindful eating, stress-busting, and rest, we're not just warding off the next cold; we're building a fortress for our long-term health.

So, as we march on to the next chapter of our gut health odyssey, let's remember: nurturing our gut flora is akin to tending to the roots of a tree, ensuring it stands tall and sturdy. Here's to a journey that enriches our years and the life within them, guiding us toward a future brimming with health and vitality.

SUMMARY AND CALL TO ACTION: YOUR PERSONAL BLUEPRINT FOR HARNESSING THE NEW FRONTIERS OF GUT HEALTH

As we've journeyed together through the bustling marketplace of microbiome research, tasting the delights of personalized nutrition, savoring the strength of probiotics, and marveling at the fusion of traditional and alternative medicine, it's clear we stand at the threshold of a new era in health and wellness. Our exploration has unveiled the intricate dance between our gut health and overall well-being and illuminated a path forward, rich with possibilities and promise.

Now, it's your turn to embark on this exciting adventure, armed with knowledge and inspired by the potential to craft a life of vitality and longevity. Here's your action plan, a roadmap to navigate this new frontier:

- **Embrace Personalized Nutrition:** Begin by listening to your body's unique needs. Reflect on how different foods make you feel, and consider consulting with a nutritionist who can help tailor your diet to your gut's microbiome. The goal is a bespoke eating plan that nourishes you, body and soul.
- **Incorporate Probiotics and Prebiotics:** Make these your gut's best friends. Whether through diet—think yogurt, kefir, sauerkraut, and high-fiber foods—or supplements,

enrich your gut flora. Pay attention to how your body responds and adjust accordingly.

- **Explore Herbal Helpers:** Venture into the garden of herbal supplements with curiosity. Start with the champions—ginger for digestion, peppermint for IBS relief, turmeric for inflammation, and psyllium husk for fiber. Always prioritize quality and consult a healthcare professional before starting any new supplement.

- **Marry Traditional and Alternative Medicine:** Open your mind to the possibilities at the intersection of conventional wisdom and alternative practices. Whether it's acupuncture for stress relief or functional medicine for a holistic health overview, seek professionals who bridge these worlds.

- **Prioritize Gut-Immune Harmony:** Acknowledge the profound connection between your gut and immune system. Adopt a lifestyle that supports this dynamic duo—balanced nutrition, stress management, and quality sleep- are your pillars.

- **Stay Informed and Engaged:** The landscape of gut health is ever-evolving.

- Keep your finger on the pulse of new research, breakthroughs, and therapies. Consider joining forums or community groups to share experiences and learn from others.

- **Document Your Journey:** Keep a health diary. Note your dietary experiments, your body's responses to different probiotics, and any changes you observe in your well-being. This record will be invaluable in understanding what works best for you.

- **Consult the Experts:** Never go it alone. Build a team of trusted healthcare providers who are knowledgeable about the latest in gut health and open to an integrative approach. Your health is a collaborative effort.

As we close this chapter and look to the horizon, remember that the journey to optimal gut health is deeply personal, filled with discovery, and uniquely yours. Embrace it with enthusiasm, armed with the wisdom gleaned from our exploration of the new frontiers of gut health. Here's to a future where we live longer and thrive with vitality, joy, and an inner ecosystem that's in harmonious balance. Let the adventure begin!

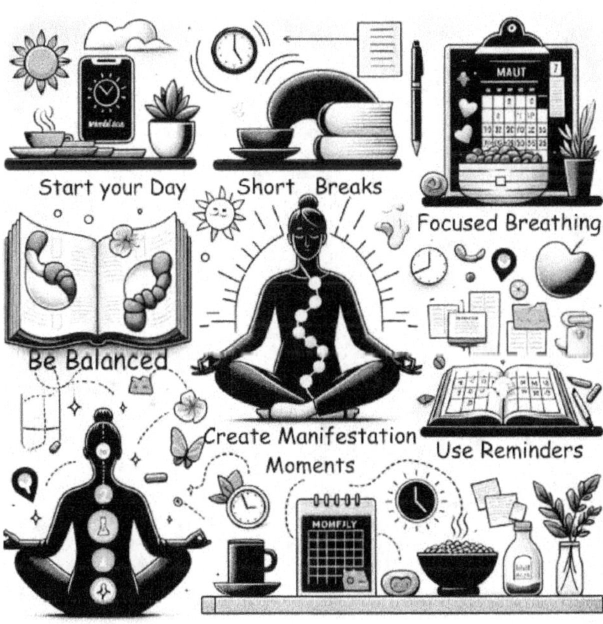

MERGING PATHS: THE CONFLUENCE OF TRADITIONAL AND ALTERNATIVE MEDICINE

Imagine yourself as a master chef in your kitchen, surrounded by a mix of classic ingredients and quirky ones you've picked up from your travels. You're about to whip up a dish that's a little bit of this and a little bit of that, aiming for a culinary masterpiece that comforts the soul while tickling the taste buds. This is akin to navigating the world of gut health, blending Western medicine's sturdy, reliable recipes with the zest and flair of alternative remedies. The goal? A custom-made health strategy that's as unique as your signature dish.

In this chapter, we'll delve into the art of combining traditional and alternative medicine to create a holistic approach to gut health. We'll explore the scientific foundations of Western medicine, from its evidence-based treatments to its proven methodologies. Alongside this, we'll introduce the vibrant and diverse world of alternative therapies—herbal remedies, acupuncture, probiotics, and more—each bringing its own unique benefits to the table.

By the end of this chapter, you'll be equipped with the knowledge to create a personalized health plan that incorporates the best of both worlds. Like a culinary masterpiece, this integrated approach to gut health will not only provide comfort and healing but also rejuvenate your overall well-being. So, let's embark on this journey together, blending the familiar with the novel, and crafting a health strategy that's as delightful and effective as your favorite dish.

8.1 THE BEST OF BOTH WORLDS: INTEGRATING TRADITIONAL AND ALTERNATIVE MEDICINE

Integrative Health Models

Consider integrative health the ultimate dinner party, where modern medicine and its alternative cousins are invited to contribute to the feast. This isn't about choosing sides; it's about creating a symphony of health, with each approach playing its part. The Functional Medicine model, for example, digs deep into the "why" behind your health hiccups, marrying traditional diagnostics with a holistic view that includes diet, lifestyle, and even your emotional landscape. It's less about slapping a band-aid on the problem and more about nurturing the whole garden, so to speak, to prevent weeds from taking over.

Benefits of Integration

Marrying traditional practices with alternative therapies brings a bounty of benefits. For one, it offers a care package that's as comprehensive as a seven-course meal. Ever felt like your doctor was just scratching the surface? This approach aims to peel back the layers, examining how everything from your snack choices to your stress levels affects your gut health. Plus, it's empowering. Understanding your health's "whys" and "hows" can inspire you to take charge, making decisions that nourish your body and soul.

Case Studies

Take the story of a lady wrestling with IBS. Conventional treatments eased her discomfort but never really got to the heart of the matter. By weaving in stress management, tweaking her diet, and introducing her to a few herbal allies, she saw her symptoms improve and felt a surge in her overall zest for life.

Or consider the gentleman plagued by acid reflux, who found relief not just in his medicine cabinet but in dietary changes, mindfulness, and a sprinkle of supplements, allowing him to dial back on the drugs and step up his quality of life.

Finding Balance

Straddling the line between traditional and alternative medicine can feel like doing a tightrope walk in a gusty wind. Here's how to keep your balance:

- **Start with Open Communication:** Chat with your healthcare provider about exploring alternative avenues. A good practitioner is your partner, not your adversary.
- **Research Thoroughly:** Dive into the evidence behind various treatments, wearing your skeptic's hat to sift through the noise and find the gems.
- **Listen to Your Body:** Tune into the feedback your body gives you. What's nourishing for one may be noxious for another.
- **Prioritize Safety:** Always loop in your healthcare team before embarking on new treatments or popping new pills, ensuring nothing clashes with your current regimen.

Sprinkle in a bit of reflection after each healthcare adventure, noting how you feel, any shifts in your well-being, and brewing questions for your next appointment. This log becomes your roadmap, guiding conversations with your care team.

Keep a treasure chest of resources—trusted websites, insightful books, and seasoned professionals in the integrative health space. This arsenal provides knowledge, keeping you informed and engaged in your health journey.

Blending the old with the new in healthcare isn't just about quelling symptoms; it's a deeper dive into understanding and actively shaping your well-being. This chapter is your compass, pointing towards a tailored approach to gut health that harmonizes the age-old wisdom of traditional medicine with the innovative spirit of alternative therapies.

8.2 HERBAL HELPERS: NATURAL SUPPLEMENTS FOR GUT HEALTH

In the grand, lush garden of Mother Nature, there's a particular corner reserved for those leafy greens and roots that have been waiting patiently to share their secret recipes for gut health. Imagine this section as the VIP lounge of nature's pharmacy, where the plants have mingled with humans for generations, offering a leaf or a root in friendship to help us digest, soothe, and thrive.

Herbal Supplements Overview

Dive into the herbal cabinet, and you'll find a world bursting with the colors, smells, and tastes of nature's remedies. From the cool zing of peppermint that can send stomach woes packing to the robust embrace of psyllium husk that sweeps through your bowels like a gentle broom, these earth-born helpers are steeped in the lore of traditional healers and the households of wise grandmothers alike. With its unique character, each herb brings a story of digestive aid that crosses continents and epochs.

Evidence-Based Benefits

Let's put our lab goggles on for a moment and peek at the evidence stacking up behind these herbal champions:

- **Ginger:** This fiery root is like the friend who always knows how to calm you down. Studies have shown it's quite the maestro at easing nausea and perking up a sluggish digestive parade, making nutrients dance into your system with greater ease.
- **Peppermint:** Not just for freshening breath, peppermint oil has been caught red-handed relaxing those pesky gut muscles that kick up a fuss during IBS concerts, helping to reduce the bloating and discomfort with a cool, minty finesse.
- **Turmeric:** Cloaked in its golden hue, turmeric is the superhero of the spice rack, wielding anti-inflammatory powers that help quell the flames of gut irritation and protect the delicate lining of our digestive tract with a curcumin shield.
- **Psyllium Husk:** The gentle giant of the fiber world, psyllium husk is the go-to for keeping things moving smoothly down the tracks, feeding the good gut bacteria, and ensuring your digestive journey is as regular as clockwork.

Safe Usage Guidelines

While these herbal allies are ready to rally to our aid, navigating their use wisely is critical to ensuring we don't end up in a pickle:

- **Consult with Professionals:** Before you start brewing teas or popping pills, having a chat with a healthcare sage or an herbalist can keep you on the right track, ensuring the herbs play nicely with any other options you're taking.

- **Quality Matters:** In the world of supplements, not all bottles are filled with the same level of enchantment. Look for reputable brands that let third parties peek behind the curtain to verify their potions are pure and potent.
- **Listen to Your Body:** Introduce new herbs gently, letting your body whisper its approval or concerns. Personalize your herbal journey based on what sings to your system.
- **Be Aware of Interactions:** Some herbs can tango too fiercely with prescription meds. For example, St. John's Wort might step on the toes of certain drugs, while ginger could turn a slow dance with blood thinners into a more complicated number.

Custom Herbal Formulations

For those yearning for a concoction tailored just to their digestive whims, custom herbal formulations are like having a couture dress made for your gut:

- **Initial Assessment:** Picture a consultation with a herbal wizard, who'll map out your digestive landscape, exploring the hills and valleys of your symptoms and health history.
- **Selection of Herbs:** With wisdom and care, a blend of herbs will be crafted for you, targeting not just the surface ripples but diving deep into the roots of your digestive tales.
- **Ongoing Evaluation:** As you embark on your herbal adventure, keeping in touch with your practitioner allows for tweaks and turns, ensuring your herbal blend is as dynamic as your life story.

This path toward gut health, paved with the leaves and roots of herbal helpers, invites us to weave the wisdom of ancient remedies with the threads of modern science. It's a journey that supports our digestive well-being and connects us more deeply with the natural world, reminding us that sometimes, the best medicine grows under our feet, ready to be discovered and embraced.

8.3 ACUPUNCTURE AND GUT HEALTH: A STROLL DOWN ANCIENT ALLEYWAYS FOR MODERN TUMMY TROUBLES

Now, let's meander through the ancient lanes of acupuncture, a practice so old it makes your family heirlooms look like recent purchases from Ikea. Acupuncture, darling, isn't just about being a human pincushion; it's about tapping into the body's healing rhythms. Think of it as the body's internal orchestra conductor, ensuring every section is in tune, especially regarding the digestive symphony.

The secret sauce of acupuncture in coddling our digestive well-being lies in its ability to tell our body's stress manager to take a hike. Tackling the body's nervous system reduces the volume of stress hormones that love to throw a wrench in our digestive works. Moreover, it gives a little pep talk to our gut motility, ensuring that the food's journey through our innards is neither a sprint nor a marathon but just the right pace, helping to wave goodbye to the likes of constipation and its unruly cousin, diarrhea.

The proof isn't just in the pudding but in the pages of some rather stodgy scientific journals, which sing praises of acupuncture's role in the digestive chorus. From the high notes of reducing IBS's belly aches to the bass of beating constipation's sluggish tempo, the evidence is as compelling as a grandmother's home remedies—only with a bit more scientific oomph behind it.

If you're pondering how to weave acupuncture into your tapestry of gut health, here's a little guide to get you started:

Initial Tête-à-Tête: Embarking on your acupuncture adventure usually kicks off with a chat more thorough than your nosiest neighbor's inquiries. An acupuncturist will dive into your health history and current gripes, tailoring their needlework to your body's unique narrative.

Regular Rendezvous: How often you visit your acupuncturist depends on how well your insides take to their ministrations. It's a bit like dating; some may find the match perfect after a few outings, while others might need a longer courtship to see results. Together, you'll sketch out a plan that serenades your digestive woes.

Harmonizing Therapies: Just as a meal is more than its main course, acupuncture shines brightest when part of a whole platter of health strategies. This can mean anything from tweaking your diet with fibers and friendly bacteria to lacing up your sneakers for a jaunt around the block while mastering the art of not letting stress steal your lunch money. Your acupuncturist can act as the maestro, orchestrating these elements into a symphony of gut health.

Keeping Tabs: Like a diary of a love affair, tracking your journey with acupuncture helps you see how far you've come, noting the crescendos and diminuendos of your digestive well-being. This diary is your script, guiding the ongoing tweaks to your treatment, ensuring the acupuncture keeps hitting the right notes.

Stepping into the realm of acupuncture for gut health is akin to rediscovering a forgotten melody—ancient yet timeless, offering a harmonious remedy to today's tummy trials. It invites us to view our bodies as landscapes of interconnected pathways, where balance isn't just a lofty ideal but a tangible state we can achieve. With a nod to tradition and an eye on the present, acupuncture opens the door to digestive harmony and well-being that resonates through our core. So, here's to exploring this path, needle by needle, towards a symphony of gut health that's been centuries in the making.

8.4 HOMEOPATHY AND THE GUT: A DAB OF THIS, A PINCH OF THAT

Now, let's tiptoe into the garden of homeopathy, where the remedies are as delicate as a lace doily, and the philosophy is as intriguing as an Agatha Christie novel. Homeopathy, my dears, is the art of healing that subscribes to the quaint notion of "like cures like." Imagine treating an upset tummy with something that, in a heftier dose, might give your gut a run for its money. It's like fighting fire with a carefully controlled backburn - a method that's as fascinating as genteel.

The Heart of Homeopathy

In the cozy parlor of homeopathy, the body is considered wise beyond its years, capable of setting itself to rights with a nudge in the right direction. This approach doesn't just give a cursory glance at your physical ailments; it also peers over its spectacles at your emotional and mental landscape. The remedies, each a bespoke concoction, are matched to your unique symphony of symptoms and prepared with a process that involves diluting shaking until, ostensibly, the water remembers what was once there.

A Sampler of Homeopathic Remedies

In the homeopathic medicine cabinet, you'll find a variety of remedies, each suited to a particular set of digestive decorums:

- **Nux Vomica:** The go-to for those who've overindulged in life's pleasures, leaving them with indigestion and a side of irritability.
- **Pulsatilla:** Perfect for the tender-hearted soul who bloats after a fling with too many rich foods, craving comfort and fresh air.
- **Arsenicum Album:** A boon for those moments when you've dined a bit too adventurously, leading to an upset stomach with an accompanying dose of anxiety and thirst for tiny sips of water.
- **Lycopodium:** For the individual whose gut feels like a balloon ready to pop, especially as the day wears into the evening.

The Great Debate

Ah, but here's where the plot thickens. The scientific salon is all aflutter with debates on homeopathy's merits. With their monocles firmly in place, critics argue that it's all a bit of smoke and mirrors, with remedies too diluted to do more than tickle. Yet, some whisper of relief was found in these gentle potions, calling for a broader conversation and deeper investigation into how these ancient practices might benefit our modern guts.

Embarking on a Homeopathic Journey

Should you decide to wander down this path, here are a few pointers to keep you straight and narrow:

- **Seek Out a Sage:** Find yourself a homeopath with a twinkle in their eye and wisdom in their heart. They'll craft a remedy as unique as your own story.
- **Gentle Beginnings:** Start with the slightest whisper of a

dose, and watch with a keen eye how your body responds. Homeopathy is a gentle nudge, not a shove.

- **Keep a Ledger**: Document your adventures in a journal. Note every twist and turn of your symptoms; this log will be your map and compass.
- **A Holistic Ensemble**: Let homeopathy be but one instrument in your health orchestra. Diet, lifestyle, and perhaps a pinch of meditation should all play their parts in your symphony of well-being.
- **Educate Yourself**: Stay curious, my dear. Read, discuss, and delve into homeopathy and gut health mysteries. Knowledge is not just power; it's empowerment.

Navigating the gentle waters of homeopathy for gut health is akin to learning a graceful dance. It's a step back into a time when healing was as much about understanding the individual as treating the ailment. While the jury may still be out in the halls of science, the tales of those who've found solace in these remedies invite us to explore with an open mind and a hopeful heart. With a blend of wisdom, caution, and a dash of adventure, homeopathy offers a genteel companion on our journey to digestive harmony.

8.5 THE POWER OF TOUCH: MASSAGE THERAPY FOR DIGESTIVE WELLNESS

Let's waltz into the somewhat overlooked ballroom of health remedies, where the power of touch takes center stage. Massage therapy, a gem with roots as ancient as any folklore, possesses a quiet power in nurturing our digestive health. It's not just about indulging in pampering; it's about unlocking a door to a more tranquil and efficient gut.

Therapeutic Massage for the Gut

Mention massage might conjure images of blissful relaxation. Yet, when it comes to our digestive ballet, a specific type of massage – let's call it the belly dance – can lead. This abdominal-focused routine involves a series of gentle, circular pressures that coax life into our sluggish intestines, easing constipation and that ever-annoying bloating. It's like having a friendly internal conversation, encouraging everything to move along as it should while ensuring the digestive orchestra has ample blood flow to play their symphony beautifully.

Benefits of Massage

Embracing massage therapy as part of your gut wellness waltz offers a bouquet of benefits:

- **Stress Reduction**: Considering our guts tend to tighten up like a knot in times of stress, the relaxation massage brings to the table (literally) helps untangle this knot, allowing for smoother digestive processes.
- **Improved Bowel Function:** For those moments when your inner workings feel more like a traffic jam, regular abdominal massages can help restore order to the chaos, guiding you back to regularity.
- **Enhanced Nutrient Absorption:** With better blood flow to the digestive organs comes a more efficient nutrient pick-up, ensuring your body reaps the total rewards of your diet.

Evidence and Practice

While some may raise an eyebrow at the thought of massage as a digestive aid, the research annals are beginning to fill with nods of approval. Studies are whispering tales of improvement in gastrointestinal symptoms post-massage, lending a scientific backing to what our bodies have known. If you're keen to introduce your gut to the healing hands of massage, seek out a therapist seasoned in the art of abdominal techniques, ensuring a beneficial and safe experience.

Self-Massage Techniques

On those days when the therapist's table is out of reach, fear not, for the art of self-massage awaits. Here's a snippet of how you can be your own masseuse:

- **Starting Position:** Find a cozy spot to lie down or sit, ensuring your abdominal area is as relaxed as an old cat in the sun.
- **Technique:** With the palms of your hands, embark on a gentle exploration of your abdomen. Picture outlining your colon – up on the right, across the top, and down on the left – encouraging your inner workings to wake and move.
- **Frequency:** A daily rendezvous of a few minutes with your abdomen can work wonders, especially if your digestive system tends to be sluggish or if stress is a frequent visitor.

Introducing massage therapy into your digestive care routine is akin to adding a spoonful of honey to your tea – sweet, soothing, and full of benefits. Whether you opt for professional sessions or dabble in self-massage, this age-old technique offers a pathway to a happier gut and a more serene state of being.

As we close the book on our exploration of gut health's alternative avenues, we've journeyed through ancient remedies, touched on the power of needles and diluted solutions, and now, the healing hands of massage. Each stop on this tour underscores the beauty of a holistic approach to our well-being, marrying the wisdom of ages with our contemporary quest for health. The road to digestive harmony is private, dotted with opportunities to tune into our bodies' needs and rhythms, discovering along the way the perfect blend of treatments that resonate with our unique constitution. Here's to a journey filled with discovery, healing, and a dash of old-fashioned wisdom, guiding us toward a life of vibrant health and joy.

YOUR ACTION PLAN FOR INTEGRATING TRADITIONAL AND ALTERNATIVE GUT HEALTH PRACTICES IN 7 EASY STEPS

Step 1: Build Your Health Team

- Identify and consult with healthcare professionals who are open to an integrative approach, including general practitioners, gastroenterologists, nutritionists, herbalists, acupuncturists, homeopaths, and massage therapists.
- Ensure these practitioners communicate and collaborate on your care plan.

Step 2: Explore and Personalize Your Treatment Options

- Research and experiment with herbal supplements that support gut health, such as ginger for nausea, peppermint for IBS, turmeric for inflammation, and psyllium husk for fiber intake.
- Consider acupuncture to address digestive issues, focusing on reducing stress and enhancing gut motility.
- Explore homeopathic remedies like Nux Vomica for indigestion, Pulsatilla for post-rich food discomfort, Arsenicum Album for food poisoning symptoms, and Lycopodium for bloating.

Step 3: Document Your Health Journey

- Keep a detailed journal of your dietary intake, symptoms, and any side effects or improvements noted from the therapies or remedies you're trying.
- Record your emotional and physical responses to treatments to help identify what works best for your unique body.

Step 4: Integrate and Balance Your Approach

- Combine dietary modifications with your chosen therapies for a holistic approach. Incorporate foods that support gut health and consider eliminating known irritants.
- Integrate stress management practices like meditation, yoga, or other relaxation techniques to support digestive health.
- Schedule regular massage therapy sessions focusing on abdominal massage to support digestion.

Step 5: Review and Adjust Regularly

- Regularly review your health journal and discuss your progress with your healthcare team to make necessary adjustments to your treatment plan.
- Be open to modifying your approach based on your body's responses and any new insights or research findings in gut health management.

Step 6: Commit to Continuous Learning and Adjustment

- Stay informed about the latest research in traditional and alternative gut health medicine.
- Attend workshops, seminars, or webinars focused on integrative health approaches to digestive wellness.

Step 7: Foster Patience and Mindfulness Throughout Your Journey

- Recognize that finding the right balance of treatments and therapies is a process that requires time, patience, and experimentation.
- Practice mindfulness and listen to your body, allowing it to guide you toward the therapies and lifestyle changes that best support your health and well-being.

By following this action plan, you equip yourself with a comprehensive strategy for exploring the confluence of traditional and alternative medicine in your quest for optimal gut health. Remember, this journey is deeply personal, and what works for one individual may not work for another. Stay curious, open-minded, and proactive in your pursuit of digestive wellness.

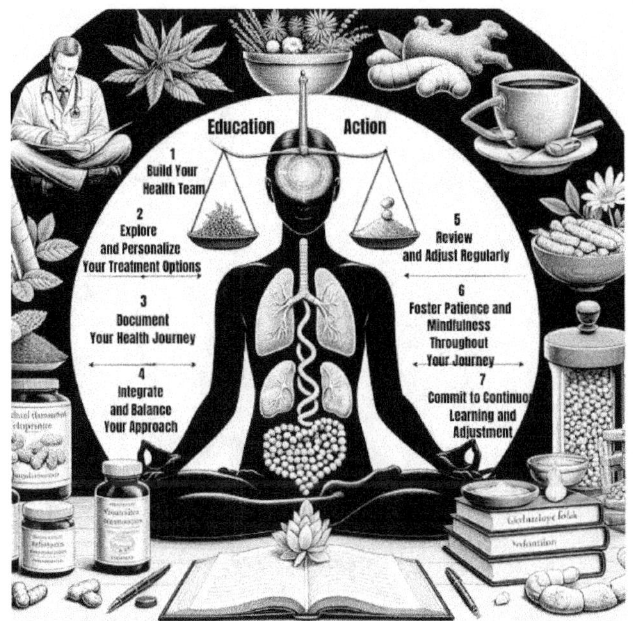
Education
Action
1
Build Your
Health Team
2
Explore
and Personalize
Your Treatment Options
3
Document
Your Health Journey
4
Integrate
and Balance
Your Approach
5
Review
and Adjust Regularly
6
Foster Patience and
Mindfulness
Throughout
Your Journey
7
Commit to Continuous
Learning and
Adjustment

GUT FEELINGS: THE SECRET CHATS BETWEEN YOUR BELLY AND BRAIN

Have you ever wondered why we say "gut-wrenching" when upset or trust our "gut feeling" when making a tough call? It's as if our everyday lingo has been dropping hints about a secret society where our gut and emotions mingle. Well, buckle up because science is finally lifting the curtain on this mystery, and let me tell you, it's more fascinating than any gossip at the bridge club or over the water cooler.

This chapter will take you on a little tour of this inner dialogue, showing how friendly your gut and mood are. It's like discovering they've been best pals since childhood, influencing each other in ways we're just starting to gab about.

THE INNER CONNECTION

It turns out our gut is more than just a food processor; it's a nerve center with more gossip lines than a busy switchboard, all thanks to the enteric nervous system. This bundle of neurons is why we often call the gut our "second brain." It's involved in everything from breaking down that tuna casserole to shaping our emotions. In short, a cheerful gut is like sunshine for your mood.

Trusting Your Gut

Those "gut instincts" aren't just old wives' tales or fodder for quirky sayings. They're the real deal, signals from the gut-brain hotline that can clue us into how we're feeling. Ever notice how a bout of nerves can send you sprinting to the loo or how being over the moon can make you not hungry at all? That's the gut-brain axis in action, showing its cards.

Creating Mind-Gut Harmony

Achieving a zen-like balance between your mind and gut might seem like a tall order, but it's all about tuning into the body's whispers (sometimes, it's loud protests). Here are some golden nuggets on how to keep the peace:

- **Mindful Munching:** Take your time with your food, savoring each bite. Pay attention to how different foods play with your emotions and gut. It's like being a detective in your kitchen.
- **Stress-Busting:** Stress wrenches our digestive harmony, so finding your chill is vital. Find what flips your relaxation switch, whether through knitting, gardening, or meditating.

Hands-On Exercises

Getting cozy with your gut feelings takes a bit of elbow grease, but it's worth the effort. Here are some exercises to put you on speaking terms with your inner self:

- **Gut Diary:** Spend a week playing detective with your gut. Jot down what you eat, how your belly feels, and what's going on in your heart and head. You might just find some patterns that make you go, "Aha!"
- **Intuition Checks:** Breathe and listen to your gut next time you're hemming and hawing over a decision. Is it doing somersaults? Sitting quietly? These clues can be your guide in the decision-making dance.

And why not spruce up your journey with some visuals, like a colorful chart of the gut-brain axis, or dive into journal prompts that get you reflecting on your gut's wisdom? It's about making this exploration insightful but a tad fun too.

Embracing the whispers and sometimes shouts from our gut opens a new avenue to emotional well-being and a more harmonious existence. This chapter is your guidebook, filled with insights, laughter, and practical tips to help you navigate the wonderful world of gut feelings. Here's to a journey of tuning in, understanding, and even having a good chuckle at the marvelous conversations happening inside us.

9.2 LAUGHTER: THE BEST MEDICINE FOR YOUR GUT

Laughter, often seen as a simple expression of joy, carries a profound ability to act as a natural stress reliever, significantly influencing our gut health. The act of laughing initiates a cascade of positive physiological changes in our bodies, directly impacting our digestive system. This section explores the multifaceted benefits of laughter on gut health and outlines practical ways to weave more laughter into our daily lives.

Laughter and Stress Reduction

When we laugh, our body's stress response is significantly damp-ened. The act of laughing decreases the production of stress hormones such as cortisol and adrenaline, which are known to affect gut function negatively. It's akin to hitting a "reset" button on our body's stress levels. As these hormones decrease, our body becomes more relaxed, fostering an environment where gut health can flourish. Beyond the immediate feeling of lightness and joy, laughter creates a chain reaction that can benefit our digestive system long-term.

Physiological Benefits

The benefits of laughter extend deep into our physiological well-being, particularly concerning our digestive health. Here's a closer look at how laughter influences our body:

- **Improved Digestion**: Laughter increases the intake of oxygen-rich air, stimulating our heart, lungs, and muscles. This increase in oxygen circulation aids digestion by ensuring our digestive organs receive the oxygen they need to function optimally.
- **Enhanced Gut Motility**: The physical act of laughing involves the contraction of abdominal muscles, which can help move contents through the digestive tract more efficiently. This gentle, internal massage aids in relieving symptoms of constipation and promoting regular bowel movements.
- **Boost in Immunity**: Laughter has been shown to activate the release of immune cells and infection-fighting antibodies, improving our body's resistance to pathogens that can upset our gut health.

Incorporating More Laughter

Integrating laughter into our daily routine can be surprisingly simple and incredibly rewarding. Here are some suggestions to help you find more reasons to laugh:

- **Laughter Yoga**: This innovative exercise combines unconditional laughter with yogic breathing (Pranayama). Practiced in groups, laughter yoga encourages eye contact and childlike playfulness, leading to genuine, contagious laughter.
- **Seek Out Humor**: Make an effort to watch a funny movie, read a humorous book, or listen to a comedy podcast. Surrounding yourself with sources of humor can naturally lead to more laughter in your life.
- **Spend Time with Friends Who Make You Laugh**: Social interactions that spark joy and laughter are invaluable. Plan regular meet-ups with friends or family members who have a knack for seeing the funny side of life.

Real-Life Stories

The impact of laughter on gut health is not just theoretical; countless individuals have experienced significant improvements in their digestive health by incorporating more laughter into their lives. Consider the story of Emily, who, after joining a local laughter yoga club, noticed a marked decrease in her IBS symptoms. The regular, hearty laughs not only helped her manage stress but also seemed to alleviate her digestive discomfort. Then there's Michael, who habitually watched comedy shows in the evening. He found that not only did his stress levels go down, but his chronic constipation also improved. These stories underscore the potential of laughter as a simple yet powerful tool in promoting gut health and overall well-being.

The exploration of laughter as a remedy for improving gut health opens up a delightful avenue for enhancing our quality of life. By understanding the intricate relationship between laughter, stress reduction, and digestion, we can harness the healing power of joy to foster a healthier gut. Through practical steps and inspired by real-life successes, we discover that laughter indeed can be the best medicine for our gut, offering a natural, enjoyable path to digestive wellness.

9.3 THE GUT-EMOTION WALTZ: STEPPING LIGHTLY AWAY FROM TROUBLESOME TWIRLS

Ah, the intricate ballet of our gut health twining with our emotions – it's a bit like a tango, wouldn't you say? Except perhaps with fewer roses between our teeth and more probiotics on our plates. This entwined dance can often lead us into a bit of a do-si-do with unwanted consequences. This chapter aims to shed light on the merry-go-round of gut-emotion interplay, which, if left unchecked, can have us spinning in circles of discomfort and dismay. With a dash of patience, a sprinkle of insight, and a good dollop of curiosity, we can explore and understand this complex relationship and find our way to a healthier, happier jig.

Cycle Explanation

Picture this: your gut health and emotional state are like an old married couple who've danced together for years. When one missteps, the other will follow, causing a tumble in the overall performance. If our gut starts to grumble – perhaps from one too many processed meals or an inflammatory comment from a friend – our mood will likely sour, leading to a cascade of emotional and digestive discomfort. This delicate balance requires a thoughtful approach, emphasizing the importance of caring for our physical and emotional well-being to keep the dance smooth and enjoyable.

Identifying Triggers

To untwist the tangle of the gut-emotion waltz, we first must determine what music is playing that sets our feet astray. This task is as personal as your secret family recipe, requiring you to tune into your rhythm and beats. Here's how to start:

- **Journaling Journey:** Keep a diary like it's the most captivating novel you've ever read. Detail your meals, gut twinges, and mood swings. Look for the plot twist – perhaps a particular food or stressor that spirals your narrative.
- **Bodily Whispers:** Pay attention to the quiet whispers of your body. It's often more articulate than we give it credit for, signaling displeasure through subtle signs like changes in appetite or mood after certain meals.
- **Stress and Solace**: Reflect on your stress levels and how you seek comfort. Stress, the stealthy saboteur, can sneak up and disrupt both gut health and emotional equilibrium.

Breaking the Cycle

Having identified what throws you off balance, it's time to choreograph a new routine:

- **Dietary Do-Over:** Let's start with the basics – your diet. Swapping processed fare for whole, fiber-rich foods can turn your health waltz into a graceful glide. Including stars like omega-3-packed salmon and probiotic-rich yogurt can also make your gut flora flourish.
- **Stress-Relief Serenade:** Incorporate stress-busting activities into your daily life. Whether it's deep breathing in a meditative moment, the gentle stretch of yoga, or

losing yourself in a hobby that fills you with joy, find your rhythm to reduce stress.

- **Helping Hands:** Sometimes, we need a dance instructor. Cognitive-behavioral therapy (CBT) and dietary guidance from professionals can provide the support and steps required to navigate the dance floor of our well-being.

Success Stories

Let's waltz through a gallery of victors who've twirled past their troubles. Anna, once entangled in anxiety and irritable bowel syndrome, cut dairy and stress from her diet, finding solace in yoga. Her journey led her from a stumbling step to a confident stride. Then there's David, whose chronic stress had him tripping over his own feet until mindfulness and a whole-foods diet restored his gut harmony and emotional balance.

Recognizing the connection between our physical and emotional states is crucial to mastering the steps of the gut-emotion waltz. By identifying triggers, embracing comprehensive strategies, and drawing inspiration from those who've danced before us, we can glide towards a future of harmonious health. Let's lace up our dancing shoes and step gracefully into a life of wellness and joy.

9.4 HEALING FROM THE INSIDE OUT: EMOTIONAL STRATEGIES FOR GUT HEALTH

Imagine your emotional wellness and gut health taking a leisurely stroll together through a peaceful park, chatting away like lifelong chums. But then life, with its endless to-do lists and calendar alerts, barges in, often leaving our insides feeling like they've been through a spin cycle. Acknowledging how our emotional world can shake up our digestive system is like unlocking a secret garden of healing and personal growth.

Emotional Wellness: A Pillar of Gut Health

Our emotions are more than just the backdrop to our daily lives; they're like the interior decorators of our gut health, for better or worse. The butterflies from an upcoming social gathering or the weight of an unsettled dispute don't just evaporate. Instead, they take up residence in our gut, stirring up trouble. Tending to our emotional garden isn't simply about feeling chipper; it's about cultivating a haven where our digestive system can flourish. When managing stress and fostering joy, we're laying the groundwork for a thriving gut.

Therapeutic Approaches: Pathways to Emotional Healing

The journey to emotional balance is peppered with various therapeutic scenic routes, each offering its unique healing viewpoint. Cognitive-behavioral therapy (CBT) and mindfulness-based stress reduction (MBSR) stand out as two promising paths, with a track record of soothing both the mind and gut by tackling emotional turmoil at its roots.

Cognitive-Behavioral Therapy (CBT): Think of CBT as a mental decluttering method that helps us sort through and toss out those gnarly thought patterns that trigger stress and anxiety. It's about switching up our mental narrative, transforming our emotional landscape, and, as a happy byproduct, easing our gut distress. CBT acts like a flashlight, exposing the mental mess that leads to emotional storms, and hands us the broom to clean it up.

Mindfulness-Based Stress Reduction (MBSR): MBSR invites us to plant our feet firmly in the now, observing our thoughts and feelings without slapping a label on them. This practice of mindfulness not only lowers stress but also has a domino effect on our gut health. Dipping our toes into mindfulness practices can usher in a tranquility that ripples through our entire being, smoothing out digestive wrinkles along the way.

Self-Care Practices: Nurturing Emotional and Gut Health

Self-care is far from a trendy hashtag; it's an essential ingredient in the recipe for a balanced life and happy gut. Here are a few self-care rituals to sprinkle throughout your day:

Journaling: There's magic in the act of transferring thoughts from mind to paper. It's a potent stress-reliever, providing clarity and insight into the emotional currents affecting our gut health. A journal can be a mirror, reflecting patterns and stressors we might overlook otherwise.

Meditation: This isn't just about hitting the pause button on life; it's about connecting deeply with ourselves. Meditation can be a powerful ally in reducing stress and fostering a serene gut environment. Even a short daily practice can improve emotional equilibrium and digestive peace.

Quality Social Interactions: The company we keep can be a tonic for our emotional and gut health. Heartfelt chats, shared laughter, and mutual support lift our spirits and can have a soothing effect on our digestive system. Nurturing positive relationships is akin to applying a soothing salve on our internal wounds.

Holistic Healing: Embracing the Whole

Healing is more than just putting a band-aid on a symptom; it's about enveloping our entire being in care and understanding. A holistic approach recognizes the intricate dance between our emotional state and physical health, especially concerning our gut. By looking at the bigger picture—how our lifestyle, thoughts, and feelings interconnect—we can uncover and address the true sources of our discomfort with tenderness and mindfulness.

As we embark on this holistic voyage, we learn the art of body listening, attuning to its whispers, and responding with gentle care. Whether through therapeutic methods, self-care rituals or simply recognizing the interplay between our emotions and gut, we're opening doors to a more unified healing process. This path not only leads to better gut health but also to a more vibrant and fulfilling existence.

Navigating the intricacies of our inner landscape, the strategies in this section light the way toward achieving emotional and gut wellness. From appreciating the crucial role of emotional well-being in our digestive health to exploring healing avenues, every step forward is a step toward glance. Through nurturing practices and a holistic outlook, we're not just treating our bodies and minds; we're healing from the inside out, paving the way to a life brimming with health and happiness.

9.5 SHARING YOUR STORY: THE THERAPEUTIC POWER OF COMMUNITY

There's something quite magical about sharing our tales in the grand tapestry of life stitched with all our triumphs and trials. It's like adding a dash of color to our canvas and those around us. Especially when we're tangled up in the complex dance between our gut health and emotional state, stumbling upon a community that gets it can feel like finding an oasis in a desert.

Community Support

Imagine you're wandering through a garden with a friend who knows every whisper of the wind and every secret of the soil. Suddenly, everything seems more vibrant, more alive. That's what finding your tribe feels like. These sanctuaries, tucked away in the corners of quaint cafes or sprawling across the digital universe, become our safe-havens. Here, our stories resonate, our voices find echoes, and the collective wisdom lights our way like a lighthouse in the gloom.

Sharing Benefits

Spinning yarns about our journeys isn't just a pastime; it's a balm for the soul. Here's why telling our tales can be as therapeutic as a cup of tea with an old friend:

- **Reduced Isolation:** Learning that others have trod similar paths weaves a fabric of belonging around us, softening the sting of loneliness that often shadows issues of gut and heart.
- **Increased Support:** When we open up, we invite not just nods of understanding but hands stretched out in support, offering solace and solutions.
- **Therapeutic Effect:** There's a certain magic in giving voice to our struggles; it can help untangle the knots in our hearts and minds, offering clarity and comfort.

Finding Your Community

Unearthing a tribe that feels like home might require some detective work, but oh, the treasures you'll find! Here's how to embark on your quest:

- **Research Online Platforms:** The digital world is brimming with nooks and crannies filled with kindred spirits. Dive into forums or social networks dedicated to gut health or emotional well-being, and listen for the sound of your own heart in the words of others.
- **Local Health Workshops:** Watch for community workshops or lectures. They're like beacons for folks walking similar journeys.

- **Wellness Centers:** These oases often host a plethora of groups, meetings, and bulletins pointing you toward local gatherings of soul mates.

Encouraging Openness

Baring your soul might seem as daunting as scaling a mountain, but the view from the top is worth it. Here are some gentle nudges to ease into sharing:

- **Start Small:** Think of your story as a tapestry. You don't have to unveil the whole masterpiece at once. Begin with a single thread.
- **Focus on Listening:** The art of active listening can throw open the doors to mutual sharing, crafting a space where trust blooms.
- **Be Authentic:** Let your true self shine through. Authenticity is contagious, inviting others to shed their masks as well.

As we weave our way through the complexities of balancing our gut health and emotional waves, the embrace of a community becomes our lighthouse, guiding us through storms. Sharing our sagas binds, heals, and lifts us, highlighting the power of togetherness in our quest for wellness. As we chart this course together, let's remember the beauty of our shared narratives and the warmth of collective understanding. These connections, these moments of mutual support, lay the foundation for a journey enriched with health and heart. They remind us that, arm in arm, we can weather any storm and savor every victory along the way.

SUMMARY, CALL TO ACTION, AND HOMEWORK ASSIGNMENT: EMBRACE THE HARMONY OF MIND-GUT WELLBEING

As we draw the curtains on our exploration of "Gut Feelings: The Secret Chats Between Your Belly and Brain," it's clear that the intricate dialogue between our emotional state and gut health is more than just idle chatter. It's a profound connection that influences our well-being in myriad ways. Each chapter has paved the way for a deeper understanding of this fascinating interplay, from the therapeutic echoes of laughter to the dance of our feelings with our gut.

Your Action Plan for Mind-Gut Harmony

- **Tune In to Your Gut:** Start by acknowledging your gut's signals daily. Whether it's a flutter of excitement or a pang of stress, recognizing these signs is the first step toward understanding the conversation happening within.
- **Foster Emotional Wellness:** Incorporate practices that enhance your emotional health, such as mindfulness or cognitive-behavioral therapy (CBT), to support your gut. Emotional balance isn't just about feeling good—it's about creating an environment where your gut can thrive.
- **Laugh More:** Embrace the healing power of laughter. Find joy in the small things, seek humor, and let laughter be a regular part of your daily life. Remember, laughter is not just medicine for the soul but also for the gut.
- **Connect and Share:** Remember to appreciate the power of community. Share your story and listen to others. Finding a support group, whether online or in-person, can provide immense comfort and understanding on your journey to gut health.

- **Practice Mindful Eating:** Pay attention to what and how you eat. Savor your meals and notice how different foods affect your feelings, emotions, and gut. This mindful approach to eating can illuminate the immediate effect of diet on your well-being.
- **Keep a Gut Diary:** For a week or more, document your meals, emotions, and gut reactions. Look for patterns and use these insights to adjust your habits for better harmony between your mind and gut.
- **Seek Joyful Movements:** Engage in activities that bring you happiness and reduce stress, be it yoga, walking, or dancing. Physical activity can improve gut motility and reduce stress-related gut issues.
- **Nurture Your Relationships:** Quality social interactions can have a soothing effect on your gut. Spend time with people who uplift you and make you laugh, reinforcing the positive loop between good company and gut health.
- **Embrace Holistic Health:** View your health through a holistic lens, recognizing the interconnection between your mental, emotional, and physical states. A comprehensive approach ensures every aspect of your well-being is noticed.
- **Stay Open and Curious:** Finally, keep an open heart and mind. Be willing to explore new practices, listen to your body, and adjust your habits as you discover what truly works for you.

As you embark on this journey toward mind-gut harmony, remember that the path is as individual as you are. What works for one may not work for another, and that's perfectly okay. The goal is not perfection but progress—toward understanding, healing, and, ultimately, a deeper connection with yourself.

Here's to your health—inside and out! Let's toast the excellent dialogue between our bellies and brains, and may we all find the balance and harmony we deserve.

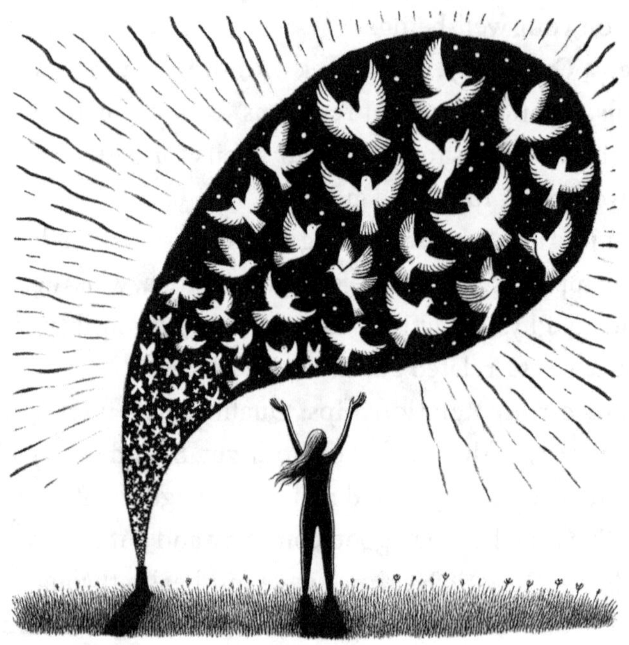

The Power of Your Words: Fueling the Journey Forward

Congratulations! You've journeyed through the twists and turns of the mind-gut connection and emerged with insights that could transform not just your life but the lives of countless others. Now, you stand at a crossroads where your experience can light the way for fellow explorers.

By sharing your thoughts and reflections on this book through an Amazon review, you do more than just voice your opinion—you become a beacon of guidance for others intrigued by the intricate dance between our guts and minds.

Your review has the power to

- Illuminate the path for others on their wellness journey.
- Encourage more curious minds to explore the wonders of the mind-gut connection.
- Spread the word about the life-changing insights this book offers.

Here's How You Can Share Your Light:

- **Reflect:** This book has influenced your understanding of the mind-gut connection. What insights resonated with you? How has your perspective changed?
- **Write:** Visit Amazon and pen down your honest review. Whether it's a newfound appreciation for your gut feelings or practical tips you've incorporated into your daily life, your unique experience matters.
- **Share:** By clicking the link below, you can directly jump to the review section and let your voice be heard. It's your chance to contribute to a growing community of knowledge-seekers.

https://shorturl.at/V77jy

Remember, your journey doesn't end here; it's just taking on a new form. By sharing your experience, you're keeping the vital conversation about the mind-gut connection alive and paving the way for others to discover their paths to wellness and understanding.

Thank you for choosing to be a part of this journey. Your willingness to share your insights brightens the flame of knowledge for everyone fascinated by the boundless possibilities of the mind-gut connection.

Together, we're not just passing on information but igniting a movement.

With heartfeld gratitude,
~Your Guide on the Mind-Gut Journey~
Cherish Dutro

REFERENCES

- Mayer, E. A., Tillisch, K., & Gupta, A. (2015). Gut/brain axis and the microbiota. Journal of Clinical Investigation, 125(3), 926–938. https://www.ncbi.nlm.nih.gov/pmc/articles/PMC4367209/

- Carabotti, M., Scirocco, A., Maselli, M. A., & Severi, C. (2018). The gut-brain axis: interactions between enteric microbiota, central and enteric nervous systems. Annals of Gastroenterology, 28(2), 203–209. https://www.ncbi.nlm.nih.gov/pmc/articles/PMC6225396/

- Foster, J. A., Rinaman, L., & Cryan, J. F. (2017). Stress & the gut-brain axis: Regulation by the microbiome. Neurobiology of Stress, 7, 124–136. https://www.sciencedirect.com/science/article/pii/S2352289516300509

- Johnson, J. (2020). Gut Health: How Deep Meditation Can Improve It. Healthline. https://www.healthline.com/health-news/gut-health-how-deep-meditation-can-improve-it

- Harvard Health Publishing. (n.d.). Healthy gut, healthier aging. Harvard Health. Retrieved March 9, 2024, from https://www.harvard.edu/staying-healthy/healthy-gut-healthier-aging

- Oklahoma Cooperative Extension Service. (n.d.). Nutrition for Older Adults: Digestion, Food Intolerance, and Nutrition. Oklahoma State University. Retrieved March 9, 2024, from https://extension.ok-state.edu/fact-sheets/nutrition-for-older-adults-digestion-food-intolerance-and-nutrition.html

- Jovanovski, E., Khayyat, R., Zurbau, A., Komishon, A., Mazhar, N., Sievenpiper, J. L., ... & Vuksan, V. (2021). Impact of dietary fiber on inflammation and insulin resistance. National Library of Medicine. https://www.ncbi.nlm.nih.gov/pmc/articles/PMC10220584/

- Vinderola, G., Ouwehand, A., Salminen, S., & von Wright, A. (2001). Probiotics and prebiotics in the elderly. PMC. https://www.ncbi.nlm.nih.gov/pmc/articles/PMC1743061/

- Dimidi, E., Cox, S. R., Rossi, M., & Whelan, K. (2021). Fermented foods as probiotics: A review. PMC. https://www.ncbi.nlm.nih.gov/pmc/articles/PMC8588917/

- Administration for Community Living. (2019). Nutrition Needs for Older Adults: Fiber.

https://acl.gov/sites/default/files/nutrition/Nutrition-Needs_Fiber_FINAL-2.19-FINAL_508.pdf

- Zeratsky, K. (n.d.). Water after meals: Does it disturb digestion? Mayo Clinic. Retrieved March 9, 2024, from https://www.mayoclinic.org/healthy-lifestyle/nutrition-and-healthy-eating/expert-answers/digestion/faq-20058348
- WiCross. (n.d.). The Truth about Food Labels: Decoding Nutritional Information and Making Informed Choices. Retrieved March 9, 2024, from https://wicross.com/food-labels/
- Valenti, J. (2021, July 12). Fermented-food diet increases microbiome diversity, decreases inflammatory proteins, study finds. Stanford Medicine News Center. https://med.stanford.edu/news/all-news/2021/07/fermented-food-diet-increases-microbiome-diversity-lowers-inflammation.html
- Lecomte, V., Kaakoush, N. O., Maloney, C. A., Raipuria, M., Huinao, K. D., Mitchell, H. M., & Morris, M. J. (2015). Changes in gut microbiota in rats fed a high fat diet correlate with obesity-associated metabolic parameters. PLoS ONE, 10(5), e0126931. https://www.ncbi.nlm.nih.gov/pmc/articles/PMC4578152/
- Link, R. (n.d.). How to Do an Elimination Diet and Why. Healthline. Retrieved March 9, 2024, from https://www.healthline.com/nutrition/elimination-diet
- Chassaing, B., Van de Wiele, T., De Bodt, J., Marzorati, M., & Gewirtz, A. T. (2021). Dietary emulsifiers directly alter human microbiota composition and gene expression ex vivo potentiating intestinal inflammation. Gut, 70(8), 1414–1425. https://www.ncbi.nlm.nih.gov/pmc/articles/PMC8011970/
- Johns Hopkins Medicine. (n.d.). Finding the Hidden Sugar in the Foods You Eat. https://www.hopkinsmedicine.org/health/wellness-and-prevention/finding-the-hidden-sugar-in-the-foods-you-eat
- Foster, J. A., Rinaman, L., & Cryan, J. F. (2017). Stress & the gut-brain axis: Regulation by the microbiome. Neurobiology of Stress, 7, 124–136. https://www.sciencedirect.com/science/article/pii/S2352289516300509 (Note: This reference appears to be a duplicate from the previous list. Please ensure to adjust as necessary.)
- Van Oudenhove, L., & Aziz, Q. (2020). The role of psychosocial stress in the pathophysiology of the gastrointestinal tract. Journal of Gastroenterology and Hepatology, 35(5), 664–673. https://www.ncbi.nlm.nih.gov/pmc/articles/PMC7219460/

- Smith, R. P., Easson, C., Lyle, S. M., Kapoor, R., Donnelly, C. P., Davidson, E. J., ... & Tartar, J. L. (2019). Gut microbiome diversity is associated with sleep physiology in humans. PLoS ONE, 14(10), e0222394. https://www.ncbi.nlm.nih.gov/pmc/articles/PMC6779243/
- WORKBLIS. (n.d.). Tai Chi for Digestive Health. Retrieved March 9, 2024, from https://www.workblis.com/tai-chi-for-digestive-health
- Monda, V., Villano, I., Messina, A., Valenzano, A., Esposito, T., Moscatelli, F., ... Messina, G. (2017). Exercise modifies the gut microbiota with positive health effects. Oxidative Medicine and Cellular Longevity, 2017. https://www.ncbi.nlm.nih.gov/pmc/articles/PMC5357536/
- GoodRx. (n.d.). 4 Benefits of Walking After Eating. Retrieved March 9, 2024, from https://www.goodrx.com/well-being/movement-exercise/benefits-of-walking-after-eating
- Ticinesi, A., Lauretani, F., Milani, C., Nouvenne, A., Tana, C., Del Rio, D., ... Meschi, T. (2023). Effects of exercise and physical activity on gut microbiota changes in the elderly: a systematic review. BMC Geriatrics, 23, Article 40. https://bmcgeriatr.biomedcentral.com/articles/10.1186/s12877-023-04066-y
- Popkin, B. M., D'Anci, K. E., & Rosenberg, I. H. (2010). Water, Hydration and Health. Nutrition Reviews, 68(8), 439–458. https://www.ncbi.nlm.nih.gov/pmc/articles/PMC2908954/
- Frontiers in Cellular and Infection Microbiology. (2023). Editorial: New techniques in microbiome research. https://www.frontiersin.org/articles/10.3389/fcimb.2023.1158392
- Cape Crystal Brands. (n.d.). The Future of Personalized Nutrition: Tailoring Diets with AI and Gut Microbiome Analysis. Retrieved March 9, 2024, from https://www.capecrystalbrands.com/blogs/cape-crystal-brands/the-future-of-personalized-nutrition-tailoring-diets-with-ai-and-gut-microbiome-analysis
- Zhang, H., DiBaise, J. K., Zuccolo, A., Kudrna, D., Braidotti, M., Yu, Y., ... Bruce, K. (2023). Synergy and oxygen adaptation for development of next-generation probiotics. Nature, 591, 66–73. https://www.nature.com/articles/s41586-023-06378-w
- National Institute on Aging. (n.d.). Unique gut microbiome patterns linked to healthy aging and increased longevity. Retrieved March 9, 2024, from https://www.nia.nih.gov/news/unique-gut-microbiome-patterns-linked-healthy-aging-increased-longevity
- Chi, L., Gao, B., Bian, X., Tu, P., Ru, H., & Lu, K. (2017). Integrative

Medicine for Gastrointestinal Disease. PMCID: PMC5605819. https://www.ncbi.nlm.nih.gov/pmc/articles/PMC5605819/

- Mego, M., Accarino, A., Tzortzis, G., Vulevic, J., Gibson, G., & Guarner, F. (2018). Prebiotic Potential of Herbal Medicines Used in Digestive Health and Disease. Journal of Clinical Gastroenterology, 52(Suppl 1), S35–S45. https://www.ncbi.nlm.nih.gov/pmc/articles/PMC6065514/

- Chao, G., Zhang, S. (2022). Acupuncture for the Treatment of Diarrhea-Predominant Irritable Bowel Syndrome. JAMA Network Open, 5(10):e2799968. https://jamanetwork.com/journals/jamanetworkopen/fullarticle/2799968

- Sinan, U., & Arslan, S. (2021). The Effect of Abdominal Massage on Gastrointestinal Functions. Complementary Therapies in Clinical Practice, 42, 101263. https://www.sciencedirect.com/science/article/abs/pii/S0965229920318203

- Mayer, E. A., Tillisch, K., & Gupta, A. (2015). Gut/brain axis and the microbiota. Journal of Clinical Investigation, 125(3), 926–938. https://www.ncbi.nlm.nih.gov/pmc/articles/PMC4367209/

- Robinson, L., Smith, M., & Segal, J. (2021). Laughter is the Best Medicine. HelpGuide. https://www.helpguide.org/articles/mental-health/laughter-is-the-best-medicine.htm

- Winch, G. (2021). 7 Ways to Break Free from a Negative Emotional Cycle. Psychology Today. https://www.psychologytoday.com/us/blog/the-freedom-change/202201/7-ways-break-free-negative-emotional-cycle

- Liang, H., Chen, C., Li, F., Wang, L., Zheng, X., Cai, Y., ... Zhang, L. (2023). Sense of community and mental health: a cross-sectional study of the correlation of sense of community with depression, anxiety, and stress. PMCID: PMC10314672. https://www.ncbi.nlm.nih.gov/pmc/articles/PMC10314672/